Emerging Issues in Family and Individual Resilience

Series Editors
Amanda W. Harrist
Stephan M. Wilson

More information about this series at http://www.springer.com/series/13415

Amanda W. Harrist • Brandt C. Gardner
Editors

Biobehavioral Markers in Risk and Resilience Research

Springer

Editors
Amanda W. Harrist
Center for Family Resilience
Oklahoma State University
Stillwater, OK, USA

Brandt C. Gardner
Department of Human Development
and Family Science
Oklahoma State University
Stillwater, OK, USA

ISSN 2366-6072 ISSN 2366-6080 (electronic)
Emerging Issues in Family and Individual Resilience
ISBN 978-3-030-05951-4 ISBN 978-3-030-05952-1 (eBook)
https://doi.org/10.1007/978-3-030-05952-1

This Springer imprint is published by the registered company Springer Nature Switzerland AG
The registered company address is: Gewerbestrasse 11, 6330 Cham, Switzerland

Preface

I teach a lot of undergraduate students at Oklahoma State University. Most of them are in lower-division classes about human development, relationship formation, and marriage. Because of that, I get a lot of personal questions from students. Rarely are they asked in front of the class (although sometimes a brave soul will venture there during a lecture). They usually happen after class or during my office hours. And they almost always start with the word "why." They want to understand themselves better: "Why do I feel this way when _________?" They want to understand a romantic partner: "Why does my partner always ____________?" I love these questions, because they are indicative of the student's desire to understand, to improve, to connect, or to help.

They are beginning to sense something that many professionals and scholars have already learned: There is power in knowing. There is power in understanding. Our students sense that. They want to know. We want to know, too. That is why many of us have entered higher education and decided to stay there. Knowing and learning is fun, rewarding, and fulfilling. We get to spend our days asking and answering those "why" questions. Some are asked by our students. Some we ask ourselves, which can then lead to a study, or a grant, or a manuscript.

I was enthused when asked to help plan the 2017 Chautauqua sponsored by Oklahoma State University, because it was an opportunity to ask some more "why" questions or, to be more accurate, to invite people to contribute who could teach us how to find answers to those "why" questions. We were able to identify some tremendous scholars working in diverse yet complementary areas who were willing to come together to share their latest work with us. It was a phenomenal conference, and I'm pleased that we are able to compile their efforts in this volume.

Historically, this conference and the accompanying volume has always been linked to resilience—the capacity of the individual or family to endure adversity or to recover following a trauma. This conference and volume are no different. We have chosen to focus on biobehavioral markers in risk and resilience, tapping into a growing body of empirical efforts to connect biological and physiological measures to behavioral and health outcomes.

For many years, the costs associated with such measures likely prevented these variables from finding their way into general human development, psychological, and sociological research. However, the pace at which technology is advancing is placing these powerful measures into the hands of a range of scholars to ask and answer meaningful questions using biological and physiological data. The proceedings of this conference provided phenomenal insight into the accessibility and utility of these new measures and approaches to the study of people and relationships.

Just a handful of months following the 2017 Chautauqua, my wife and I were notified of the sudden death of our daughter, Paiton. She had been preparing for her sophomore year at the University of Utah when she unexpectedly passed away in her sleep. There followed many of those "why" questions. The physicians and medical examiners had very little in the way of answers for us.

The days, weeks, and months that followed posed a supreme test to our family's resilience. No longer was this a theory or a concept to be defined or debated. It was real, and it was all about our survival as a family. There was no comfort to be found in the academic theories, nor in the empirical findings of a research study. There were things happening within our bodies that affected how we felt, that affected what we did. Some I understood, but much I didn't.

We did find comfort in our relationships, both with each other and with people outside our family. This event brought out both the best and the worst in people. Some, who we never would have expected to lean on in such a time, were incredibly helpful and insightful and knew exactly what we needed—even when we did not. Others, who we might have expected to be a source of encouragement or support, turned out to be the opposite. We learned much about ourselves and about others during that time. We did our best to marshal our strength to do the things that needed to be done, to get by.

We are better now, remarkably better, all things considered. As I reflect upon that experience—which is ongoing—I see better than I did before the relevance of the "why" questions. Before, they were cute, curious things sometimes asked by students who wanted to learn a little more about themselves. Or they were interesting questions that might lead me to my next publication. Now, I see the "why" questions as a tool by which we try and make meaning of the world around us. It is our admitting that there is an answer that we desperately want or even need that is just beyond our reach.

I believe the scholarship in this volume will place some of these answers within reach. It will inspire students who want to get a glimpse at where the social and behavioral sciences are headed in the future. It will empower established scholars who may be looking for examples of forward-thinking approaches to utilizing these measures in their study of human behavior and relationships. It will also serve as a model for how researchers of all types might incorporate an interdisciplinary approach to their study of the human experience.

Ultimately, whatever our research interests might be, and however we choose to investigate those interests, all of us are seeking to improve the lives of our fellow human beings. We are trying to shed light on the unknown. We are trying to answer the "why" questions in life. I hope this volume spurs readers onward in that quest.

Stillwater, OK, USA

Amanda W. Harrist
Brandt C. Gardner

Acknowledgments

Oklahoma State University's Center for Family Resilience (CFR) hosts an annual *Chautauqua: A Conference on Family Resilience*. The goals of the conference are (a) to bring together distinguished and rising scholars from diverse disciplines to discuss cutting-edge work focused on one annual theme within the broader area of family resilience research and (b) to foster a translational approach within the study of resilience, such that practical applications for family health and well-being can be developed from basic resilience research. This includes development of action steps in conjunction with community stakeholders. The papers presented at each year's Chautauqua are the core of the chapters that comprise the respective volumes in our Emerging Issues in Family and Individual Resilience series.

We would like to thank those involved in planning and hosting the 2017 Chautauqua. These include CFR doctoral student interns Jillian Bailey, Ashley Harvey, and Amy Huffer and Mary Gardner, who helped with the local arrangements and Authors' Dinner. Thank you most especially to Brooke Tuttle and Tia Claybrook, who were in charge of many of the details of conference planning and implementation. We are also appreciative of HDFS's Accountant Rita Ryan, who coordinated financial issues, and Associate Dean Dr. Christine Johnson, whose staff took care of the registration.

We are extremely grateful to the following OSU Center Directors who helped fund the 2017 Chautauqua that made this volume possible: Dr. Michael Merton for the CFR; Dr. Jennifer Hays-Grudo for CIRCA, the Center for Integrative Research on Childhood Adversity; and Dr. Amy Payton for IBEaR, the Institute for Building Early Relationships. Thank you also to Dr. Sissy Osteen, HDFS Department Head, for her financial support of the Chautauqua.

For the preparation of this volume, we are indebted to our editor, Jennifer Hadley, who is consistently patient and supportive. Thank you also to the CFR's Shania Ramos for doing the indexing for each chapter and to CFR Research Associates Drs. Lucia Ciciolla, Michael Criss, Julie Croff, Catherine Curtis, Amanda Morris, Mike Stout, Amy Tate, and John Walker, who reviewed the chapters (sometimes twice). They also conducted interviews and wrote the narratives summarized in this volume's breakout boxes that provide such meaningful application and advice to professionals in each chapter. These couldn't have been included without the willingness of the community professionals and families who participated in the interviews, for which we are very grateful.

Finally, we acknowledge and dedicate this volume to the many individuals and families who face significant risk every day and wish for them resilience.

Contents

Contributors

Clint L. Broadbent, Ph.D. Department of Human Development and Family Science, Oklahoma State University, Stillwater, OK, USA

Department of Teacher Education & Family Development, Southern Utah University, Cedar City, UT, USA

Jennifer Byrd-Craven, Ph.D. Department of Psychology, Oklahoma State University, Stillwater, OK, USA

Nikki Clauss, M.A. Department of Psychology, Oklahoma State University, Stillwater, OK, USA

H. Harrington Cleveland, Ph.D. Department of Human Development and Family Science, The Pennsylvania State University, University Park, PA, USA

Brandt C. Gardner, Ph.D. Department of Human Development and Family Science, Oklahoma State University, Stillwater, OK, USA

Amanda M. Griffin, Ph.D. University of Oregon, Eugene, OR, USA

Nathan Hardy, Ph.D. Department of Human Development and Family Science, Oklahoma State University, Stillwater, OK, USA

Bridget E. Hatfield, Ph.D. College of Public Health and Human Sciences, School of Social and Behavioral Health Sciences, Oregon State University, Corvallis, OR, USA

Pilyoung Kim, Ph.D. Department of Psychology, University of Denver, Denver, CO, USA

Julie H. Marino, Ph.D. Department of Surgery, University of Oklahoma School of Community Medicine, Tulsa, OK, USA

University of Oklahoma Integrative Immunology Center, Tulsa, OK, USA

Theodore F. Robles, Ph.D. Department of Psychology, University of California, Los Angeles, Los Angeles, CA, USA

Gabriel L. Schlomer, Ph.D. University at Albany, State University of New York, Albany, NY, USA

Todd A. Spencer, Ph.D. Department of Human Development and Family Science, Oklahoma State University, Stillwater, OK, USA

Elizabeth J. Susman, Ph.D. Department of Biobehavioral Health, The Pennsylvania State University, University Park, PA, USA

T. Kent Teague, Ph.D. Department of Surgery, University of Oklahoma School of Community Medicine, Tulsa, OK, USA

Department of Pharmaceutical Sciences, University of Oklahoma College of Pharmacy, Tulsa, OK, USA

Department of Biochemistry and Microbiology, Oklahoma State University Center for the Health Sciences, Tulsa, OK, USA

University of Oklahoma Integrative Immunology Center, Tulsa, OK, USA

Rebekah Tribble, M.S. Department of Psychology, University of Denver, Denver, CO, USA

David J. Vandenbergh, Ph.D. Department of Biobehavioral Health, The Pennsylvania State University, University Park, PA, USA

Institute of the Neurosciences, The Pennsylvania State University, University Park, PA, USA

About the Editors

Amanda W. Harrist received her Ph.D. in Child and Family Studies from the University of Tennessee, Knoxville. She is currently a Professor of Human Development and Family Science at Oklahoma State University, where she is also Associate Director for Education and Translation at the Center for Family Resilience and Core Director of Human & Community Research Training Core for the Center for Integrative Research on Childhood Adversity. Her research is focused on understanding psychosocial risk and protective processes in children's social contexts, particularly the parent-child relationship and peer relations at school.

Brandt C. Gardner received his Ph.D. in Marriage & Family Therapy from Texas Tech University. He is currently an Associate Professor of Human Development and Family Science at Oklahoma State University. He spends the majority of his professional time teaching about and studying communication processes and interaction dynamics in marital and couple relationships.

Stephan M. Wilson is a Ph.D. graduate in Child and Family Studies from the University of Tennessee, Knoxville. He is an NCFR Fellow, Fulbright Fellow, and Regents Professor at Oklahoma State University, has received Legend Recognition from the American Association of Family and Consumer Sciences, and has numerous teaching, research, and community engagement recognitions. His areas of expertise include cross-cultural family science and adolescent social competence.

Chapter 1
The Immune System as a Sensor and Regulator of Stress: Implications in Human Development and Disease

Julie H. Marino and T. Kent Teague

The purpose of this chapter is to describe how stress influences the interplay between the immune system and the neuroendocrine system and how chronic stress can lead to long-lasting maladaptation. For more technical and in-depth reading on this topic, we recommend the following review articles: (Dantzer, O'Connor, Freund, Johnson, & Kelley, 2008; Glaser & Kiecolt-Glaser, 2005; Miller & Raison, 2016). We will discuss how a stressful environment during early development influences epigenetics. We will also review how stress-induced immune dysregulation can culminate in disease states, specifically mood disorders.

J. H. Marino
Department of Surgery, University of Oklahoma School of Community Medicine, Tulsa, OK, USA

University of Oklahoma Integrative Immunology Center, Tulsa, OK, USA
e-mail: julie-marino@ouhsc.edu

T. K. Teague (✉)
Department of Surgery, University of Oklahoma School of Community Medicine, Tulsa, OK, USA

Department of Pharmaceutical Sciences, University of Oklahoma College of Pharmacy, Tulsa, OK, USA

Department of Biochemistry and Microbiology, Oklahoma State University Center for the Health Sciences, Tulsa, OK, USA

University of Oklahoma Integrative Immunology Center, Tulsa, OK, USA
e-mail: kent-teague@ouhsc.edu

A. W. Harrist, B. C. Gardner (eds.), *Biobehavioral Markers in Risk and Resilience Research*, Emerging Issues in Family and Individual Resilience,
https://doi.org/10.1007/978-3-030-05952-1_1

1.1 Perceptions and Old Friends

Imagine one of our early human ancestors living in a primitive environment as a hunter/gatherer. He routinely dealt with danger from predators and infectious pathogens. These were his most intense and life-threatening stressors. What did he need to survive? What were the evolutionary pressures on him and the thousands of generations that followed? Obviously, the survival advantage went to those who developed rapid response mechanisms in the brain to perceive and avoid danger coupled with a robust immune system to fend off infection. An important point here is that perceived danger needed to be immediately dealt with regardless of whether or not the danger turned out to be real. The mechanisms that evolved to deal with perceived danger still exist within us today, even though most of us live lives with far less frequent life-threatening encounters. When a predator is chasing you, there is no time to wait to figure out if the predator will successfully lacerate you and open you to infection. The defense mechanisms need to be turned on immediately, regardless of later cost. The systems that have evolved are even more complex as the story does not just involve us and the pathogens and predators. We are not only made of human cells but instead are filled and covered with a diverse microbiome. As Miller and Raison detailed in their review "The role of inflammation in depression: From evolutionary imperative to modern treatment target," humans did not evolve in these inflammatory environments alone but instead co-evolved with immunoregulatory organisms they refer to as "old friends" (2016).

The brain's response to perceived stress is famously referred to as the "fight or flight" response and has been widely studied (reviewed in Kozlowska, Walker, McLean, & Carrive, 2015). Classically we think of the "flight or fight" response as the physiological call to action that involves activation of the HPA axis and the sympathetic nervous system and its communication hormones such as epinephrine (adrenaline) and norepinephrine (reviewed in Goligorsky, 2001); all of this is an effort to avoid danger. Yet within the last couple of decades this primitive survival response has been shown to directly engage the immune system (reviewed in Dhabhar, 2014). Psychological stressors are now known to elicit an immune response similar to the way specific pathogens demand a specific immune reaction (reviewed in Miller & Raison, 2016). It makes sense that this would be the case, if indeed our immune reactions evolved from ancestral times to react to risk perception and not just infections after they happen. Miller and Raison refer to this as "inflammatory bias" or the tendency to skew an organism toward the activation of inflammatory pathways after induced stress. In more traditional rural environments, this stress is episodic and is hypothesized to be kept in balance by minimally pathogenic organisms that push the immune response back toward an anti-inflammatory state when the stressful encounters are resolved (Miller & Raison, 2016).

Today, this bias takes on other aspects as we are no longer subject to the same evolutionary pressures that existed in the lives of our ancestors. We live in an environment of perpetual "perceived threats" and thus chronic stress ensues. Disease states related to autoimmunity, allergy, and inflammation have skyrocketed as society has become more urbanized (Haahtela et al., 2013). The "old friends" or microorganisms and parasites common to more rural environments that helped to balance our immune system by keeping inflammatory pathways in check did not evolve for this very different environment and neither did we. As the global population has shifted toward city dwellers, humans have increasingly lost contact with these "old friends," resulting in a population of "exacerbated inflammatory bias" which is impacted by new stressors (Miller & Raison, 2016).

1.2 Emergence of the Field of Psychoneuroimmunology

The immune system encompasses the components that an organism uses to protect itself against infection and to repair tissue damage. These components include specialized cells, tissues, and chemical messengers that gear up an organism to ward off infectious threats. This defense system can be divided into two main categories—innate immunity and adaptive immunity. Innate immunity is the first line of defense that includes basic barriers to infection such as the epithelium and the mucosal membranes and cells that elicit inflammatory responses to immediate threats. Adaptive immunity is a more highly evolved system of specialized cells such as T cells and B cells that can respond to immunological challenge by initiating specific antibody secretion (humoral response) or directly destroying infected cells (cellular response) and ultimately is responsible for the immune system remembering previous infections.

The neuroendocrine system uses the hypothalamus and the pituitary and adrenal glands (HPA axis) to control stress hormone production. It is a complex system that regulates growth, development, metabolism, behavior, reproduction, blood pressure, and numerous other biological functions. The interactions between the immune system, the sympathetic nervous system, and the endocrine system are pronounced when an individual encounters an emotional or environmental stressor (Segerstrom & Miller, 2004). Psychoneuroimmunology, a term coined by Robert Ader and Nicholas Cohen in 1975, is the field that studies these complex interactions (Ader & Cohen, 1975).

Differentiating between acute and chronic stress is important as they ultimately may lead to distinct physiological outcomes. Acute stress can be classified as stress that lasts for an hour or less. When acute stress activates the hypothalamic-pituitary adrenal axis and the sympathetic nervous system, the resulting "stress cascade" (reviewed in Miller & O'Callaghan, 2002) directly affects immune responses. Acute stress activates or heightens the body's first line of defense (Dhabhar, 2009a, 2009b) (innate immunity-driven inflammation) which buys the body time to fend off and assess the danger and respond more specifically later. If the threat turns out to be real and dangerous, the adaptive arm of immunity will be activated to provide long-term specific protection from the stressor. If the threat is not real, the system will normally recover and go back to its original state. As described above, this makes sense from an evolutionary standpoint. Early humans on the hunt with a triggered flight or fight response would have the advantage of having their immune system primed for a more rapid response if they were wounded or otherwise injured while seeking food sources (Miller & Raison, 2016).

Chronic stress induced by long-term, repetitive insults lasting weeks, months, or even years may engage the same processes as acute stress, however, often without sufficient recovery time between episodes. Modern humans tend to live with constant pressures at work and at home, often for their entire lives. Many of these stressors are perceived as normal; however, if stress persists in this way, the body eventually adapts (as described in the epigenetic section below) and the normal immune response becomes dysregulated, leading to weakened immunity or autoimmunity. One way the body adapts is by becoming insensitive to cortisol via glucocorticoid receptor resistance (Cohen et al., 2012). Loss of normal feedback inhibition can lead to or exacerbate depression and other diseases (reviewed in Tsigos, Kyrou, Kassi, & Chrousos, 2000). Because stress activates inflammatory cytokines in the innate immune system (Miller, Maletic, & Raison, 2009), a person under chronic stress may live in a slightly "inflammatory state." For example, it has been shown that stressful childhood environments lead to increased inflammatory cytokine production in teens (Miller, Chen, & Parker, 2011). This pattern also appears in older adults showing exaggerated inflammatory cytokine expression patterns in response to life stress (Slavich & Irwin, 2014).

Living in a constant inflammatory state does not come without cost. Persistent activation of the HPA axis and subsequent glucocorticoid release accelerates some aging processes. An example in the immune system can be found in the production of new T cells. The thymus (the organ that produces T cells) atrophies during normal human development; however, in distressed individuals the atrophy occurs at a quicker rate resulting in significant decreases in the T cell compartment of the immune system (Bauer, 2013). This is an important loss because T cells are vital for effective vaccine responses and responses to viral infections and cancer.

The physiological response to stress is a uniquely individual experience. That which induces chronic stress in one person may barely register as a stressor in another. The concepts of individual and group "resilience" are fundamental to current research (Southwick, Vythilingam, & Charney, 2005) because it is important to determine what makes an individual or group more or less susceptible to different types of stress and whether or not this can be manipulated. Past trauma, age, obesity, chronic diseases, and numerous other factors that influence a person's immune status likely greatly influence their ability to deal with stress. In a meta-analysis of more than 300 articles dealing with the association of human psychological stress and the immune system, Segerstrom and Miller (2004) reported that the immune effects varied according to the kind of event (trauma vs. loss). Subjective reports of stress generally did not associate with immune change. In some cases, physical vulnerability as a function of age or disease also increased vulnerability to immune change during stressors (p. 601).

Breakout Box 1.1: Focus on Practice

Earlier in my career, I studied stress in immunology and saw the detrimental effects it had on laboratory mice. However, in my current practice as an obstetrician, I have seen the impact that stress can have on the mother as well as the baby. If a mother is stressed, she may find herself unable to keep doctor visits. One common malady from stress in pregnancy is hypertension. A hypertensive patient might find that they have stopped working or caring for other children to be on bed rest. This can cause problems in loss of income due to missing work or finding care for the other children. In addition to the problems with the mother, stress may cause the baby to be subject to pre-term delivery, early separation of the placenta or low birth weights. All in all, stress makes the mothers and babies sicker. These outcomes usually result in longer hospital stays for the mother and/or the baby, which makes the cost of care increase. There are other costs too, if the mother is hospitalized, it can take her away from other family members or time with the new baby. This has a trickle-down effect of increased morbidity and mortality. Unfortunately, maternal mortality has been creeping upward in the United States. This is why it is so important for mothers to have both physical and emotional support so that she can be maintaining her health to avoid adverse pregnancy outcomes.

—*Dr. Samuel Taylor, M.D.*

Because people do not tend to be able to gauge their stress levels very accurately and the system is very complex, we need objective biomarkers to assess individual levels of chronic and acute stress and their effects on immunity.

1.3 Stress-Induced Epigenetic Effects on the Immune System

The neuropsychiatric influence on the immune system has been documented throughout the human life span, including the prenatal, infant, childhood, teenage, middle age, and geriatric periods (Graham, Christian, & Kiecolt-Glaser, 2006). Crosstalk between the immune system and the neuroendocrine system begins with modification of gene expression (epigenetics) in utero. Instead of changing an organism's DNA, epigenetics allows early environmental changes to alter gene expression in compensatory ways (Turner, 2009). Effectively, the environment can turn on or off specific genes leading to lifelong genetic perturbations. This, in turn, can impact how a person deals with stress. For example, Weaver et al. (2004) demonstrated with rats that maternal grooming behavior toward offspring can alter HPA stress responses in their pups through methylation-dependent promoter changes in the expression of the glucocorticoid receptor in the hippocampus. Attentive mothers had offspring that had lower HPA responses to stress due to epigenetic receptor changes, and inattentive mothers raised offspring with exaggerated stress responses through the HPA. Interestingly, during the critical first week of life, the stress response could be reversed by "cross-fostering" pups born to inattentive mothers to attentive mothers (Weaver et al., 2004).

Controlled studies of alcoholism have yielded evidence of further epigenetic alterations related to stress (Stephens & Wand, 2012). Alcohol exposure during both the prenatal period and during early postnatal development leads to gene expression changes governed by histone covalent modifications and DNA methylation status (Krishnan, Sakharkar, Teppen, Berkel, & Pandey, 2014). Brain-derived neurotrophic factor (BDNF) transmits messages from neurons across the synapses. Expression of this molecule has been shown to vary during both chronic and acute stress. Stress-induced BDNF epigenetic changes can drive both anxiety and alcohol seeking behaviors (Krishnan et al., 2014). FKBP5 is an accessory component of the glucocorticoid receptor. This chaperone molecule is vulnerable to childhood trauma resulting in genetic changes that can heighten cortisol responses in traumatized individuals. This DNA modification predisposes individuals to stress-related psychiatric disorders (Klengel & Binder, 2015) and because it changes cortisol responses, undoubtedly impacts immune responses.

Epigenetic changes that occur *in utero* are likely adaptations driven by events the mother's immune and neuroendocrine systems interpret to indicate a harsh environment for the baby. These epigenetic changes may provide a survival advantage but also appear to predispose to pathologies later in life (Varriale, 2014). For example, immune activation in pregnant mice leads to sweeping changes in neuron development and activity and signal transduction in the immune system in their offspring. These changes can be traced back to epigenetic changes in histone acetylation in the glutamate receptor signaling pathway. The adult behaviors that these prenatally challenged animals exhibit mimic human models of schizophrenia (Tang, Jia, Kast, & Thomas, 2013).

1.4 Stress, the Immune System, and Mental Illness

The body of literature delineating the evidence of prenatal risks leading to mental disease has recently rapidly expanded and now presents a convincing case. For example, infants whose mothers experienced high anxiety during pregnancy had suppressed adaptive immune responses to the Hepatitis B vaccine at 6 months of age (O'Connor, Moynihan, & Caserta, 2014). Maternal influenza (Parboosing, Bao, Shen, Schaefer, & Brown, 2013) and anemia (Nielsen, Meyer, & Mortensen, 2016) have been linked to schizophrenia. Undernourishment in pregnant women has been implicated in the development of major affective disorder in their offspring and the risk for generalized anxiety disorders has been in part attributed to maternal stress and toxin exposure during prenatal development (Morgese & Trabace, 2016).

Perhaps one of the most prominent intersections of stress, the immune system, and mental illness is found in studies of mood disorders. Mood disorder diagnoses have become increasingly common in the United States (Hidaka, 2012). The statistics are sobering for this set of diseases which encompasses bipolar and major depressive disorder as almost 10% of the US population will have a mood disorder in any given 12-month period. The risk is also pronounced during childhood with a lifetime prevalence of 14% for 13–18-year-olds (Kessler, Merikangas, & Wang, 2007). Treatments have provided significant relief for many of these patients; however, up to 30% remain symptomatic after standard treatments.

A few decades ago, evidence emerged that the immune system was involved in the etiology of mood disorders (Maes, 1995; Maes, Smith, & Scharpe, 1995). This was a profound paradigm shift in both the fields of psychiatry and immunology. The brain was no longer viewed as an absolutely off-limits immune-privileged organ but instead to be subject to the effects of peripheral lymphocytes and inflammatory cytokines (Maes et al., 2009). Chronic stress is very likely linked to depression in certain individuals. Much like during infection or tissue damage, stress activates the innate immune system, triggering release of inflammatory cytokines, acute phase proteins, chemokines, and adhesion molecules. This in turn leads to disruptions in neuroendocrine function, monoamine metabolism, synaptic activity, and regional brain activity. If inflammation becomes chronic, there is a subset of individuals who are then put at higher risk for mood disorders such as depression and bipolar disorder (Muneer, 2016).

Interestingly, the normal immune response to infection induces a state termed "sickness behavior" that looks remarkably like depression (Dantzer et al., 2008). The inflammatory cytokines produced during a response to an infection signal back to the brain to alter behavior. This is a protective mechanism for the infected individual and possibly the family to conserve energy and avoid further contact. Sickness behavior is characterized by fatigue, social withdrawal, depressed mood, anorexia, and altered sleep. This set of symptoms can be induced in approximately one-third of patients who are treated with the cytokine interferon-α (Dantzer et al., 2008). It is now clear that inflammatory cytokine administration can induce the symptoms of depression and other mood disorders, further strengthening the notion that maladaptation of the immune response could lead to mental health disorders.

1.5 Conclusion

1.5.1 Future Directions

Immunology provides unique tools to assess developmental stress leading to disease. Inflammatory pathway cytokines that have been implicated in stress-related disease states, such as IL6, TGFβ, IL-10, IL-1, and TNF, can be quantified, potentially giving real-time measurements of physiological stress states. Likewise, inflammation profiles for acute phase responses like C-reactive protein can also give valuable data on an individual's susceptibility to inflammatory diseases. Even relatively simple tests such as determining shifts in T-regulatory cells in the blood have shown promise as indicators of immune dysregulation in stressed individuals (Freier et al., 2010; Ronaldson et al., 2016). Evidence has already emerged that we can predict an exaggerated inflammatory response in certain individuals (Slopen, Kubzansky, & Koenen, 2013). The next step will be harnessing these predictive indicators into preventative strategies. This may be particularly important in the prodromal phases of psychiatric illness, possibly providing a window in which to intervene with immunology based strategies.

1.5.2 Implications for Resilience

Stress induces dynamic changes in the human body that can lead to significant changes in human development and disease. Immune system and neuroendocrine responses that were once a survival advantage for early humans have turned out to be problematic for humans in urbanized cultures. For example, immune system dysregulation induced by modern society's chronic stressors leads to a higher risk for the development of mood disorders.

This begs the question: Should we use immune and neuroendocrine system monitoring and epigenetics to routinely assess individuals in stressful environments from early development through adulthood? We believe that the field of immunology can provide empirical tools to assess an individual's risk for maladaptation to stress. Early interventions can improve resilience; they may prove vital in slowing or preventing the progression of susceptible individuals in the development of stress-related diseases. Immune system profiling may offer unique insights especially into the effects of chronic stress. Importantly, these immune and neuroendocrine biomarkers can be conveniently assayed in blood or saliva throughout an individual's lifespan with minimal risk.

As we have moved from broader therapies to personalized treatments in the cancer field, so it is tantalizing to imagine this type of shift occurring at the interface of psychiatry and immunology. Genetics combined with immune system and neuroendocrine response profiling might lead us to better understand why some individuals are resilient and others more at risk for maladaptation to stress. Finally, because of the complexities of the environmental interactions, we also need to introduce social determinants of health variables into the emerging psychoneuroimmunology models in order to translate these findings in the future into meaningful interventions.

Questions for Thought and Discussion

1. Summarize the "old friends" theory.
2. What does the inflammatory bias look like in modern society and how might it look in future generations?
3. What is the interplay between stress and epigenetics?
4. Discuss the risk factors for the development of mood disorders and how immune monitoring might be used to control or alleviate the symptoms of mood disorders.

References

Ader, R., & Cohen, N. (1975). Behaviorally conditioned immunosuppression. *Psychosomatic Medicine, 37*, 333–340.

Bauer, M. E. (2013). The role of stress and adrenal hormones in immunosenescence. In J. A. Bosch, A. C. Phillips, & J. M. Lord (Eds.), *Immunosenescence, psychosocial and behavioral determinants* (pp. 221–239). New York, NY: Springer. https://doi.org/10.1007/978-1-4614-4776-4_13

Cohen, S., Janicki-Deverts, D., Doyle, W. J., Miller, G. E., Frank, E., Rabin, B. S., & Turner, R. B. (2012). Chronic stress, glucocorticoid receptor resistance, inflammation, and disease risk. *Proceedings of the National Academy of Sciences United States of America, 109*, 5995–5999. https://doi.org/10.1073/pnas.1118355109

Dantzer, R., O'Connor, J. C., Freund, G. G., Johnson, R. W., & Kelley, K. W. (2008). From inflammation to sickness and depression: When the immune system subjugates the brain. *Nature Reviews Neuroscience, 9*, 46–56. https://doi.org/10.1038/nrn2297

Dhabhar, F. S. (2009a). A hassle a day may keep the pathogens away: The fight-or-flight stress response and the augmentation of immune function. *Integrative and Comparative Biology, 49*, 215–236. https://doi.org/10.1093/icb/icp045

Dhabhar, F. S. (2009b). Enhancing versus suppressive effects of stress on immune function: Implications for immunoprotection and immunopathology. *Neuroimmunomodulation, 16*, 300–317. https://doi.org/10.1159/000216188

Dhabhar, F. S. (2014). Effects of stress on immune function: The good, the bad, and the beautiful. *Immunologic Research, 58*, 193–210. https://doi.org/10.1007/s12026-014-8517-0

Freier, E., Weber, C. S., Nowottne, U., Horn, C., Bartels, K., Meyer, S., Hildebrandt,Y., Luetkens, T., Cao, Y., Pabst, C., Muzzulini, J., Schnee, B., Brunner-Weinzierl, M. C., Marangolo, M., Bokemeyer, C., Deter, H. -C., Atanackovic, D., (2010). Decrease of CD4+FOXP3+ T regulatory cells in the peripheral blood of human subjects undergoing a mental stressor. Psychoneuroendocrinology 35(5):663–673

Glaser, R., & Kiecolt-Glaser, J. K. (2005). Stress-induced immune dysfunction: Implications for health. *Nature Reviews Immunology, 5*, 243–251.

Goligorsky, M. S. (2001). The concept of cellular "fight-or-flight" reaction to stress. *American Journal Physiology Renal Physiology, 280*, F551–F561.

Graham, J. E., Christian, L. M., & Kiecolt-Glaser, J. K. (2006). Stress, age, and immune function: Toward a lifespan approach. *Journal of Behavioral Medicine, 29*, 389–400. https://doi.org/10.1007/s10865-006-9057-4

Haahtela, T., Holgate, S., Pawankar, R., Akdis, C. A., Benjaponpitak, S., Caraballo, L., … Change World Allergy Organization Special Committee on Climate Change and Biodiversity. (2013). The biodiversity hypothesis and allergic disease, World Allergy Organization position statement. *World Allergy Organization Journal, 6*, 3.

Hidaka, B. H. (2012). Depression as a disease of modernity, explanations for increasing prevalence. *Journal of Affective Disorders, 140*, 205–214. https://doi.org/10.1016/j.jad.2011.12.036

Kessler, R. C., Merikangas, K. R., & Wang, P. S. (2007). Prevalence, comorbidity, and service utilization for mood disorders in the United States at the beginning of the twenty-first century. *Annual Review of Clinical Psychology, 3*, 137–158. https://doi.org/10.1146/annurev.clinpsy.3.022806.091444

Klengel, T., & Binder, E. B. (2015). FKBP5 allele-specific epigenetic modification in gene by environment interaction. *Neuropsychopharmacology, 40*, 244–246. https://doi.org/10.1038/npp.2014.208

Kozlowska, K., Walker, P., McLean, L., & Carrive, P. (2015). Fear and the defense cascade: Clinical implications and management. *Harvard Review of Psychiatry, 23*, 263–287. https://doi.org/10.1097/HRP.0000000000000065

Krishnan, H. R., Sakharkar, A. J., Teppen, T. L., Berkel, T. D., & Pandey, S. C. (2014). The epigenetic landscape of alcoholism. *International Review of Neurobiology, 115*, 75–116. https://doi.org/10.1016/B978-0-12-801311-3.00003-2

Maes, M. (1995). Evidence for an immune response in major depression: A review and hypothesis. *Progress in Neuro-Psychopharmacology & Biological Psychiatry, 19*, 11–38. https://doi.org/10.1016/0278-5846(94)00101-M
Maes, M., Smith, R., & Scharpe, S. (1995). The monocyte-T-lymphocyte hypothesis of major depression. *Psychoneuroendocrinology, 20*, 111–116. https://doi.org/10.1016/0306-4530(94)00066-J
Maes, M., Yirmyia, R., Noraberg, J., Brene, S., Hibbeln, J., Perini, G., … Maj, M. (2009). The inflammatory & neurodegenerative (I&ND) hypothesis of depression: Leads for future research and new drug developments in depression. *Metabolic Brain Disease, 24*, 27–53. https://doi.org/10.1007/s11011-008-9118-1
Miller, A. H., Maletic, V., & Raison, C. L. (2009). Inflammation and its discontents: The role of cytokines in the pathophysiology of major depression. *Biological Psychiatry, 65*, 732–741.
Miller, A. H., & Raison, C. L. (2016). The role of inflammation in depression: From evolutionary imperative to modern treatment target. *Nature Reviews Immunology, 16*, 22–34. https://doi.org/10.1016/j.biopsych.2008.11.029
Miller, D. B., & O'Callaghan, J. P. (2002). Neuroendocrine aspects of the response to stress. *Metabolism, 51*, 5–10. https://doi.org/10.1053/meta.2002.33184
Miller, G. E., Chen, E., & Parker, K. J. (2011). Psychological stress in childhood and susceptibility to the chronic diseases of aging: Moving toward a model of behavioral and biological mechanisms. *Psychological Bulletin, 137*, 959–997. https://doi.org/10.1037/a0024768
Morgese, M. G., & Trabace, L. (2016). Maternal malnutrition in the etiopathogenesis of psychiatric diseases: Role of polyunsaturated fatty acids. *Brain Sciences, 6*, 24. https://doi.org/10.3390/brainsci6030024
Muneer, A. (2016). Bipolar disorder: Role of inflammation and the development of disease biomarkers. *Psychiatry Investigation, 13*, 18–33. https://doi.org/10.4306/pi.2016.13.1.18
Nielsen, P. R., Meyer, U., & Mortensen, P. B. (2016). Individual and combined effects of maternal anemia and prenatal infection on risk for schizophrenia in offspring. *Schizophrenia Research, 172*, 35–40. https://doi.org/10.1016/j.schres.2016.02.025
O'Connor, T. G., Moynihan, J. A., & Caserta, M. T. (2014). Annual research review: The neuroinflammation hypothesis for stress and psychopathology in children—developmental psychoneuroimmunology. *Journal of Child Psychology & Psychiatry, 55*, 615–631. https://doi.org/10.1111/jcpp.12187
Parboosing, R., Bao, Y., Shen, L., Schaefer, C. A., & Brown, A. S. (2013). Gestational influenza and bipolar disorder in adult offspring. *JAMA Psychiatry, 70*, 677–685. https://doi.org/10.1001/jamapsychiatry.2013.896
Ronaldson, A., Gazali, A. M., Zalli, A., Kaiser, F., Thompson, S. J., Henderson, B., … Carvalho, L. (2016). Increased percentages of regulatory T cells are associated with inflammatory and neuroendocrine responses to acute psychological stress and poorer health status in older men and women. *Psychopharmacology (Berl), 233*, 1661–1668. https://doi.org/10.1007/s00213-015-3876-3
Segerstrom, S. C., & Miller, G. E. (2004). Psychological stress and the human immune system: A meta-analytic study of 30 years of inquiry. *Psychological Bulletin, 130*, 601–630. https://doi.org/10.1037/0033-2909.130.4.601
Slavich, G. M., & Irwin, M. R. (2014). From stress to inflammation and major depressive disorder: A social signal transduction theory of depression. *Psychological Bulletin, 140*, 774–815. https://doi.org/10.1037/a0035302
Slopen, N., Kubzansky, L. D., & Koenen, K. C. (2013). Internalizing and externalizing behaviors predict elevated inflammatory markers in childhood. *Psychoneuroendocrinology, 38*, 2854–2862. https://doi.org/10.1016/j.psyneuen.2013.07.012
Southwick, S. M., Vythilingam, M., & Charney, D. S. (2005). The psychobiology of depression and resilience to stress, implications for prevention and treatment. *Annual Review of Clinical Psychology, 1*, 255–291. https://doi.org/10.1146/annurev.clinpsy.1.102803.143948
Stephens, M. A., & Wand, G. (2012). Stress and the HPA axis, role of glucocorticoids in alcohol dependence. *Alcohol Research, 34*, 468–483.

Tang, B., Jia, H., Kast, R. J., & Thomas, E. A. (2013). Epigenetic changes at gene promoters in response to immune activation in utero. *Brain Behavior and Immunity, 30*, 168–175. https://doi.org/10.1016/j.bbi.2013.01.086

Tsigos, C., Kyrou, I., Kassi, E., & Chrousos, G. P. (2000). Stress, endocrine physiology and pathophysiology. In L. J. De Groot, G. Chrousos, K. Dungan, K. R. Feingold, A. Grossman, J. M. Hershman, C. Koch, M. Korbonits, R. McLachlan, M. New, J. Purnell, R. Rebar, F. Singer, & A. Vinik (Eds.), *Endotext*. South Dartmouth, MA: mdtext.com.

Turner, B. M. (2009). Epigenetic responses to environmental change and their evolutionary implications. *Philosophical Transactions of the Royal Society of London B: Biological Sciences, 364*, 3403–3418. https://doi.org/10.1098/rstb.2009.0125

Varriale, A. (2014). DNA methylation, epigenetics, and evolution in vertebrates, facts and challenges. *International Journal of Evolutionary Biology, 2014*, 475981. https://doi.org/10.1155/2014/475981

Weaver, I. C., Cervoni, N., Champagne, F. A., D'Alessio, A. C., Sharma, S., Seckl, J., ... Meaney, M. J. (2004). Epigenetic programming by maternal behavior. *Nature Neuroscience, 7*, 847–854. https://doi.org/10.1038/nn1276

Chapter 2
The Psychobiology of Family Dynamics: Bidirectional Relationships with Adrenocortical Attunement

Jennifer Byrd-Craven and Nikki Clauss

2.1 Attunement

Humans have a unique set of characteristics that distinguish us from our closest relatives. Some primary distinguishing characteristics include an elongated developmental period requiring extensive parental investment, an intense focus on social relationships, and aptitude for deciphering social information (Flinn, Quinlan, Ward, & Coe, 2007; Hrdy, 2009). Living in social groups requires the development of complex social-cognitive skills, as they are not innate and are sensitive to social and cultural context (Bretherton & Munholland, 2008; Byrne & Whiten, 1988). Given the inherent complexity of navigating social relationships in long-term social hierarchies, the prolonged human developmental period likely evolved to meet the demand to acquire social skills, and its plasticity reflective of ever-changing social pressures (Geary & Bjorklund, 2000). The human stress response appears to be uniquely suited to aid in these developmental calibrations (Del Giudice, Ellis, & Shirtcliff, 2011). Human infants have a stress response system that heavily depends on caregivers to regulate it, and experiences with caregivers up or down regulate an individual's physiological and behavioral response to stressors and challenges (Flinn, Nepomnaschy, Muehlenbein, & Ponzi, 2011; Gunnar & Donzella, 2002). Both human infants and caregivers have a suite of behaviors intended to influence each other, behaviorally and physiologically (Out et al., 2010, 2012), resulting in each partners' behavior and physiology being reciprocally influenced (Bornstein, 2009).

Adrenocortical attunement, the coordination or synchrony in the activity of the stress response systems of individuals in close relationships, is an index of biobehavioral exchange and plays a distinctive role in infant and child development.

J. Byrd-Craven (✉) · N. Clauss
Department of Psychology, Oklahoma State University, Stillwater, OK, USA
e-mail: jennifer.byrd.craven@okstate.edu; nikki.clauss@okstate.edu

A. W. Harrist, B. C. Gardner (eds.), *Biobehavioral Markers in Risk and Resilience Research*, Emerging Issues in Family and Individual Resilience,
https://doi.org/10.1007/978-3-030-05952-1_2

Yet, we know little about how attunement operates within families, including fathers' influence on attunement, particularly in families living in adverse conditions. In the following sections, we will outline the nature of close relationships in humans, with a focus on the behavioral and physiological interplay in these relationships. We will then review the impact of early experiences on the establishment of thresholds for stress response systems' activation and recovery. Finally, the role of stress response system attunement within social relationships and the development of socio-cognitive competencies will be discussed, with particular attention being given to its potential role in determining health, behavioral outcomes, and resilience to adversity.

2.2 Nature of Close Relationships and the Hypothalamic-Pituitary-Adrenal (HPA) Axis

As stated above, humans are an intensely social species who are highly motivated to form discerning and enduring bonds. This attachment is deeply rooted phylogenetically and widely distributed due to selection pressures. For example, humans have adapted to group living and form deep social bonds as a primary solution to the evolutionary problems of reproduction and survival. As such, social relationships are vital resources for managing environmental demands. Indeed, the absence of social ties has a noxious effect on health and is associated with a heightened risk for disease and early mortality (Taylor & Gonzaga, 2006; Uchino, Uno, & Holt-Lunstad, 1999). Further, human infants, compared with other primates, are exceptionally skilled at detecting and gaining investment from mothers and other caregivers. At the same time, human mothers are more discriminating in their investment (Hrdy, 1999). This forms the basis for a relatively novel mother–offspring relationship in which infants are closely monitoring their caregivers and adjusting their own behavior and physiology in accordance to the behavioral cues of their partner. The attachment system is likely the primary mechanism by which this occurs.

There are mechanisms for attachment that do not require high level cognitive or emotional functioning, and it has been recently demonstrated that babies may be born with the ability to recognize faces, even before they have ever seen their first face (Reid et al., 2017). This provides further evidence for the importance of social bonds. Such bonds are particularly essential in early life, as they set the framework for infant emotional development, and shape one's capacity to regulate stress and arousal. The formation of affiliative bonds requires coordination between the physiological states and interactive behavior of each partner (Feldman, 2007). This coordination is referred to as synchrony, which describes the process by which hormonal, physiological, and behavioral cues are exchanged between two individuals (especially parent and child) during social contact (Feldman, 2012).

The biological mechanism primarily responsible for biobehavioral synchrony is the hypothalamic-pituitary-adrenal (HPA) axis. The HPA axis is one of the two stress response systems (the autonomic nervous system being the other; see Munk et al., 1984), and it is made up of three main endocrine glands: the hypothalamus, the pituitary, and the adrenal glands, that feed into and back upon each other. In response to a stressor, the hypothalamus releases corticotropin-releasing hormone (CRH) and arginine vasopressin (AVP), which act on the anterior pituitary gland. Upon stimulation from CRH and AVP, the anterior pituitary releases adrenocorticotropic hormone (ACTH). The adrenal gland, stimulated by ACTH, then releases cortisol. In this cascade of events, there is then inhibitory activity in the prefrontal cortex, known as the negative feedback loop, that then typically prevents the potential damaging effects of continued cortisol release (Sapolsky, Romero, & Munk, 2000; Pruessner et al., 2010). There is evidence from rodent research suggesting that chronic stress disrupts the ability of the prefrontal cortex to inhibit continued release (Cerqueira, Mailliet, Almeida, Jay, & Sousa, 2007).

Cortisol is necessary for survival. However, in circumstances where cortisol is chronically elevated or poorly regulated, it can have deleterious health effects, such as neuronal death, and immune suppression. Despite these potential costs, retaining responsiveness in the HPA system ensures social learning, sharing emotions, promotes bonding, focuses attention, and enhances learning in some domains (Del Giudice et al., 2011; Shirtcliff et al., 2009). In other words, it facilitates the ability to effectively manage opportunities and threats, and reflects a sense of openness to information, principally social information (Ellis & Boyce, 2008; Flinn, 2006). Cortisol, then, can function to adaptively pattern behavior to the demands of a fluid social environment (Del Giudice et al., 2011; Huether, 1998). Its sensitivity to selectively responding to psychosocial factors makes it an excellent system for studying psychosocial development, as it can be seen as an index of which psychosocial factors have covaried with adaptive outcomes in previous generations. Humans, however, are not born with fully mature HPA systems. During the extended period of development (e.g., from birth throughout childhood), experiences play a major role in shaping basal rhythms and reactivity of the HPA system. Thus, the HPA system is under strong social regulation in infancy and early childhood, and experiences during this time can lead to permanent changes in its functioning.

The HPA axis is a system that reflects the result of adaptive trade-offs, and is, thus, vital to the study of life history traits. Life history theory (LHT) establishes a framework to study how organisms allocate finite energy across their lifespan, primarily between somatic effort (e.g., growth, immune system functioning) and reproductive effort (e.g., mating effort or parenting effort) (Stearns, 1992). It is capable of explaining the large diversity of life histories between species, but can also predict multiple life history trajectories within a species, including humans (Hill & Kaplan, 1999). Life history traits most commonly studied include size at birth; rate of maturation; age and size at maturity and reproduction; the quantity, size, and sex ratio of offspring; amount of investment in offspring; reproductive span; and length of life. Under this framework, organisms allocate their energy in a way that best maximizes or potentially best maximizes their fitness. Since energy and resources are finite, organisms are faced with a series of trade-offs throughout their lifespans, and develop life history strategies as a result. Life history strategies are combinations of life history traits and the environmental events acting upon them, and can be classified as "fast" or "slow." A fast life history strategy is characterized by rapid growth and maturation, earlier reproduction, higher quantity production of offspring, lower investment in each offspring, and a short lifespan. Fast life history strategies are common in environments with high mortality rates and low or unpredictable access to resources. A slow life history strategy, on the other hand, is associated with a stable environment with access to resources and is characterized by slower growth, delayed maturation, later reproduction, fewer offspring that are heavily invested in, and a longer lifespan (Stearns, 1977). Due to its role in energy allocation and phenotypic plasticity, the HPA axis yields information regarding how individuals are encoding aspects of their environment and adjusting behavioral strategies accordingly.

2.3 Early Experiences and HPA Functioning

As discussed above, the HPA system is exceptionally plastic over the course of development, serving to adjust this system to the demands of an unpredictable social world, as the largest source of variation in many social species is social dynamics (Geary, 2005). Early parent–offspring dynamics in a number of species, from rats to humans, appear to calibrate the HPA system (Ellis et al., 2006; Hofer, 1994; Meaney, 2001) and adjust cognitive and behavioral strategies accordingly (Belsky, Steinberg, & Draper, 1991; Del Giudice, 2009; Ellis, McFadyen-Ketchum, Dodge, Pettit, & Bates, 1999; Moffit, Caspi, & Belsky, 1992). One such relevant dynamic, and one associated with survival, growth, and health, is the predictability of maternal support.

2.3.1 Influence of Maternal Behavior

Both human and non-human research has demonstrated that the quality of maternal care or investment during the early postnatal period influences both the threshold for responding and recovery time of the stress response system (Caldji et al., 1998; Essex et al., 2002; Francis & Meaney, 1999; Liu et al., 1997; Lupien et al., 2009; Meaney, 2001). In rodents, high quality maternal care typically entails frequent bouts of nursing and high-energy maternal behaviors such as arched-back, or kyphotic, nursing and extensive licking and grooming of pups (Meaney, 2001; Moore & Power, 1992). Offspring of mothers high on these behaviors showed increased glucocorticoid feedback sensitivity, reduced corticosterone response to acute stress, and lower fearfulness in novel contexts (Liu et al., 1997), and this may reflect a phenotype that is more selective in its activation of the HPA system.

The human analog of this area of research typically examines disruptions in maternal responsiveness and positive affect, which are linked with low quality, less sensitive maternal care, and alterations in infant and child HPA reactivity. Children of depressed mothers have altered HPA responses to stressors compared to children of non-depressed mothers, and these effects have been shown even when controlling for heritability effects (Essex et al., 2002; Lupien et al., 2009), demonstrating that maternal responsiveness results in modifications to the child's HPA system, presumably preparing them for unpredictable and uncontrollable social dynamics. Outside of parental psychopathology per se, children have been shown to react to their social environment and adjust the responsiveness of the HPA system, their behavior, and their social cognitions to best suit their current social environment. In particular, the quality of family dynamics and the associated stressors appear to influence internal working models of social relationships and later social behavior. Environments that include unstable parental relationships, unpredictable or limited child investment, and insecure attachment to caregivers are often associated with a collection of traits and behaviors that bear the hallmark features of adaptive calibration of brain regions involved in social decision-making (Del Giudice et al., 2011). Individuals developing in such environments often show less trust in social relationships, girls are more likely to experience early menarche (though the mechanisms are currently being debated), engage in sexual activity at a younger age, have unstable pair bonds themselves, show limited investment in their own children, and have more children overall (Belsky et al., 1991; Byrd-Craven, Geary, Vigil, & Hoard, 2007; Vigil, Geary, & Byrd-Craven, 2006; but also see footnote[1]). Physiologically, persistent family stressors change the threshold for HPA activation, resulting in either hyper- or hypo-responsive neural pathways, which in turn, may be associated with many of the behavioral and social dynamics listed above (e.g., unstable pair bonds) (Flinn et al., 2011).

2.3.2 *Influence of Paternal Behavior*

Much less research has been conducted on the influence of the quality of paternal investment, though fathers are an implicit and important part of the social context in which the child develops and are capable of influencing the development of HPA reactivity (Geary & Flinn, 2002). Findings in this area mirror those examining harsh developmental environments overall. The most extensively studied feature of paternal investment is lack thereof, or father absence. Time spent with father in the early years of life (typically measured as the first 7 years) and mother–father relationship quality are associated with the timing of a suite of traits related to important social behaviors and life history traits such as age of menarche, age of first sex,

[1] It should be noted that these effects may be limited to industrialized, Western countries (see Sheppard, Snopkowski, & Sear, 2014), indicating that there may be novel pressures in these environments.

age of first childbirth, educational attainment, number of children, and number of reproductive mates (Byrd-Craven et al., 2007), as discussed above. In addition to time spent together, the quality of the relationship matters, as it does with mothers, but in many cases paternal effect exert their effects over and above maternal relationship influences. For example, warm father–daughter relationships are associated with delayed menarche and sexual activity (Ellis et al., 1999), a tendency toward monogamy and high investment in their own children (Del Giudice, 2009), and lower morning cortisol levels and reduced reactivity to peer stressors (Byrd-Craven, Auer, Granger, & Massey, 2012). On the other hand, father absence and associated factors (e.g., maternal stress, the presence of a step-father or maternal boyfriend) are associated with earlier menarche and onset of sexual behavior (Ellis, 2004; Surbey, 1990). These early family dynamics appear to lay the groundwork for later behavior and perceptions of social relationships, though some individuals may be more predisposed or genetically sensitive toward these early environmental features (Figueredo et al., 2006).

2.4 Adrenocortical Attunement and Developmental Outcomes

Adrenocortical attunement, or synchrony in the responding of the HPA system between individuals, is built off of work with affect contagion (Hatfield, Cacioppo, & Rapson, 1993), findings within the mirror neuron system (Iacoboni et al., 1999), and autonomic system synchrony (e.g., heart rate), which demonstrated that interaction partners coordinate their physiological responses (Kaplan, Burch, & Bloom, 1964). More recently, this has been demonstrated in a number of dyad types, prominently including mother–infant dyads. For example, Waters and colleagues examined affect contagion and associated physiological coordination in mothers and their infants after mothers had either experienced a stressful negative-evaluation, positive-evaluation, or non-stressful control task. Though they examined the autonomic nervous system rather than HPA axis activity, the infant's physiology was coordinated with their mother's physiology in all three conditions, demonstrating that infants were keenly aware of their mother's physiological state, and using it as a means of adapting their own physiology correspondingly (Waters, West, & Mendes, 2014).

Physiological synchrony, and adrenocortical attunement in particular, appears to reflect behavioral sensitivity to a social partner and is inherently bidirectional (or multi-directional) in nature. This is likely attributable to the HPA system's sensitivity to psychosocial factors. Adrenocortical attunement demonstrates how groups of individuals are processing the social context together, and because it is outside of conscious control, yet influenced by the social context, can provide a non-biased indicator of sensitivity or connectedness within the relationship. While it is beyond the scope of this chapter, it has been demonstrated in a variety of close relationships, including marital dyads. Attunement over the course of the day has been associated with time spent together (Papp, Pendry, Simon, & Adam, 2013), supporting the view that it may reflect dual information processing. Synchrony during conflict discussions is related to marital relationship quality, especially for husbands, suggesting that it may be an important index of investment in the relationship (Beck, Pietromonaco, DeBuse, Powers, & Sayer, 2013; Liu et al., 2013).

Mother–infant interactions are among some of the most important experiences that influence the development of the HPA system (Hofer, 1987). Indeed, beginning in early pregnancy and through the first year of life, infants must experience synchrony between their own physiology and behavior and the mothers' body, physical presence, and sensory cues for optimal social and emotional growth (Hrdy, 1999). This synchrony is referred to as biobehavioral attunement, as there are behavioral and biological aspects of synchrony involved. This biobehavioral attunement is reflected in many domains developmental psychologists typically study. Attunement has been consistently linked to positive child outcomes such as attachment security, language acquisition, and maturity of object play (Bigelow et al., 2010). This sharing of biological rhythms between the members of the dyad paves the way for the power of synchrony within early relationships to influence the way the social environment is shared with a significant other later in development (Feldman, 2007).

Granger and colleagues (1998) have presented evidence that the HPA axis plays a role in the dynamic mother–child biobehavioral exchange such that maternal behavior and cortisol levels are associated with their child's adrenocortical activity. Indeed, adrenocortical attunement is a biological measure that reflects behavioral sensitivity to a social partner (Hibel, Granger, Blair, & Finegood, 2015). Specifically, levels of cortisol are synchronized within a dyad or a larger group. This synchrony is bidirectional, and it demonstrates how groups of individuals are processing social context together. Although influenced by social context, adrenocortical attunement is outside of conscious awareness. Thus, it is a non-biased indicator of sensitivity or connectedness within a relationship, and HPA attunement is related to relationship quality.

Maternal postpartum behaviors are the behavioral building blocks of synchrony. Mothers regulate child physiology for better and for worse, as both positive and negative maternal behaviors impact child physiology and attunement (Blair & Raver, 2012). Positive maternal behaviors include such behaviors as: high-pitched vocalizations (often referred to as "motherese") and vocal congruence (Beebe, Alson, Jaffe, Feldstein, & Crown, 1988), exaggerated facial expressions, affective display, proximity position, body tone and movements, and affectionate touch (Levine, 2002). Maternal behaviors are coordinated with specific infant neurobehavioral sensitivities to these cues (Fleming et al., 1999). Over time, the autonomic, neurological, and endocrinological systems in each partner are sensitized to the temporal patterns of the other, leading to the formation of a unique bond. Therefore, anything that can impact these postpartum behaviors can also impact mother–infant synchrony or bonding.

While maternal behaviors are genetically programmed to some extent, they are also open to environmental influences and cultural meaning systems (Keller et al., 2003). Thus, a mother's own early life experiences can impact attunement between her and her child. For example, daughters of more sensitive, responsive mothers are also more sensitive and responsive to their own offspring. Because attunement is affected by maternal quality, maternal quality is transmitted across generations. Animal studies have demonstrated that this phenomenon is often due to epigenetics. Like humans, rats display individual differences in maternal care that appear to be passed down from mother to offspring in a stable manner. Champagne and Meaney (2001) found that maternal care quality is dependent on estrogen sensitivity in the medial preoptic area (mPOA), and a female's estrogen sensitivity in the mPOA depends on the quality of maternal care she received.

Whether an infant is born pre-term or full-term may also have an impact on synchrony. Premature birth is correlated with higher maternal depression and decreased infant alertness (Field, 2002). As previously described, the parent–infant relationship is shaped, in part, by parental behavior, and depressed mothers tend to display less maternal behaviors. However, infant behavior can also shape synchrony. Premature infants are less socially responsive and generally less alert than full-term infants due to their neurological immaturity, and therefore described as less rewarding social partners (Eckerman, Oehler, Hannan, & Moliter, 1995). Therefore, premature infants often experience less synchrony with mothers and fathers (Feldman, 2007). Indeed, Feldman and Eidelman (2007) found that infant–mother and infant–father synchrony could both be predicted by infant autonomic maturity level (as measured by cardiac vagal tone), in addition to postpartum behavior.

There is ample evidence for the existence and importance of adrenocortical attunement between mothers and their infants, but less is known about father–infant attunement. What is known is that social affiliation is probably a pre-requisite for paternal behavior in mammals (Wynne-Edwards & Reburn, 2000). If the father is an invested partner, their hormonal profile is similar to the maternal hormonal profile directly before their child is born (Storey, Walsh, Quinton, & Wynne-Edwards, 2000). For example, male plasma prolactin and estradiol levels increase while testosterone and cortisol levels decrease before childbirth, which is the hormonal profile necessary for several maternal behaviors. Fathers' hormonal response patterns to infants appear to be moderated by the quality of the man's relationship with the child's mother (Geary & Flinn, 2002; Storey et al., 2000). Men with more tentative pair bonds to their partner and who interact infrequently with their infants do not show these changes. High quality pair bonds are associated with more paternal investment in both modern and traditional hunter-gatherer cultures (Quinlan, 2003).

Given this, it is not surprising that the limited evidence available on attunement in fathers suggests that father–child attunement is dependent on the level of attunement between the father and the mother (Saxbe et al., 2014). Additionally, adrenocortical synchrony between husbands and wives is highly dependent on the level of investment of the husband and, subsequently, the amount of time the husband spends with his wife (Papp et al., 2013). It also appears as though the more support a mother receives from the father of her children, the more sensitive of a parent she is. This increase in maternal behaviors associated with paternal support is also associated with lower child cortisol responses to mildly challenging situations (Clauss, Byrd-Craven, Kennison, & Chua, 2018). Thus, invested fathers clearly play a role in their child's HPA axis functioning. Further evidence for this is that the fathers' parenting style is associated with toddler cortisol responses to challenge (Mills-Koonce et al., 2011) and to adolescent girls' adrenocortical responses to peer interactions (Byrd-Craven et al., 2012). Perhaps their role in the development of their child's HPA axis function contributes to the association between father–child bonding, father–mother relationship, and the timing of life history traits in offspring. Children from low-stress families who have spent sufficient time with their fathers during their first 7 years of life tend to follow slower life history trajectories (Ellis et al., 1999). This may include later onset of several biological events and behaviors associated with reproduction, as discussed above, such as menarche, age of first sex, and age of first pregnancy as well as educational attainment (Byrd-Craven et al., 2007).

2.5 Sex Differences

There is mounting evidence that girls and boys are, on average, differentially susceptible to developmental stressors, with most studies showing boys as more at risk for a variety of negative developmental outcomes, from conception to death (Geary, 2016). The full scope of these differences is beyond the focus of this chapter. We focus here on sex differences that have the potential to impact adrenocortical attunement with caregivers. Externalizing behaviors, more common in boys than in girls, appear to influence physiological synchrony. Boys with higher externalizing behaviors show disrupted parent–child co-regulation of respiratory sinus arrhythmia (RSA), an index of parasympathetic nervous system activity. This is coupled with the fact that boys, on average, depend more on the regulatory support from caregivers than do girls (Weinberg, Tronick, Cohn, & Olson, 1999), and may explain why boys are more susceptible to many developmental stressors.

Breakout Box 2.1: Implications for Practice

My clinical experience includes 8 years of work with victims of domestic violence and 17 years of working with high-risk youth and their families. My work has not focused on physiological attunement between parents and children. However, I have noticed a dynamic among families exposed to chronic stress as it often is manifested physically in similar ways for mothers and children. For example, women and the children in their custody who are victims of domestic violence often are symptomatic when they are forced to be in contact with the abusers. Although the abuser may have left the home, the family often must have ongoing contact with the abuser either through the court system or during exchanges of the children if there is visitation. Many times, my clients and their children develop digestive issues (e.g., diarrhea) and resulting dehydration before, during, and after these interactions with the abuser. My clients also develop fatigue and migraine headaches after particularly intense sessions in which they "took to their beds," emotionally and physically exhausted from the therapy session. Likewise, children often report stomachaches and being tired during periods of stress. These physiological manifestations often have been exacerbated in my low-income mothers who tend to work in physically demanding environments which often leads to chronic pain. In addition, I suspect a lack of healthcare and paid sick leave contributed this. If you can't afford to take time off work for an injury, you're going to work through it making things worse. This is mirrored in children who miss many days of school due to illness often without proper health care. The daily stress of struggling to meet basic needs can result in depression, anxiety, and more frequent physical health symptoms. I often saw my clients' age in front of my eyes over the period of months. In sum, you have often seen a form of synchronization regarding how mothers and their children cope with chronic stress. Unfortunately, this cycle often continues as most mothers are not in a healthy position to help their children because of their own situation.

—Machele Anderson, LPC

There are well-known effects of maternal depression on mother–infant interaction and maternal sensitivity (discussed above). There is evidence to suggest that the greater male sensitivity to variations in caregiving is prominent in male infants of depressed mothers (Carter, Garrity-Rokous, Chazan-Cohen, Little, & Briggs-Gowan, 2001; Murray, Kempton, Woolgar, & Hooper, 1993), and these differences have been observed as early as 3 months (Weinberg, Beeghly, Olson, & Tronick, 2008). Mothers with a history of abuse show different patterns of adrenocortical attunement with sons compared to daughters. Non-maltreated mothers showed more attunement with their infant daughters, whereas mothers with a history of maltreatment showed more attunement with their sons. This suggests that the stress response system is one mechanism for the trans-generational transmission of adverse experiences, and that this may differ by sex (Fuchs, Mohler, Resch, & Kaess, 2016). Taken together, these findings suggest that boys and girls elicit different patterns of mutual responsiveness from their caregivers.

2.6 Individual Differences

As much as the HPA system appears to selectively respond to psychosocial factors within the environment for humans overall, there are individual differences in the pattern and intensity of this responding. These underlying differences encompass genetic, temperamental, and neurobiological factors that predispose some individuals to being more vulnerable to negative, harsh, or unpredictable environments, as well as more likely to benefit from positive, supportive environments (Boyce & Ellis, 2005). In particular, genes identified as contributing to these vulnerabilities are involved in serotonergic and dopaminergic pathways, both of which have deep connections with the stress response systems (Belsky & Pluess, 2013; Del Giudice, 2015). More focally, animal studies demonstrate that maternal behavior influences expression of glucocorticoid receptors, fundamentally altering offspring's sensitivity to their environment (see Szyf, Weaver, Champagne, Diorio, & Meaney, 2005). Epigenetic regulation of glucocorticoid receptors has also been shown to be responsive to human parental behavior. For example, a history of child abuse was found to be associated with altered glucocorticoid receptor expression in victims of suicide compared with controls, suggesting a common substrate of responsiveness to maternal care and individual differences across species (McGowan et al., 2009). Taken together, these findings suggest that those with genetic predispositions especially sensitive to context may be most likely to attune to their caregivers, for better or worse, and may be more impacted by lack of caregiver behavioral and physiological regulation.

Temperament also has genetic underpinnings and has been shown to impact behavioral and physiological synchrony between infants and caregivers. Infant–mother adrenocortical attunement has been shown to be lower for highly reactive children, and this lack of attunement is consistent across time. Temperament characteristics also interact with attachment stress. In these contexts, infant surgency is associated with higher infant cortisol overall, contributing to lack of mother–infant attunement (Hibel et al., 2015). Relatedly, negative infant temperament (e.g., demanding, fussy, highly reactive) is associated with increased maternal depression and lower maternal sensitivity (Tester-Jones, O'Mahen, Watkins, & Karl, 2015), demonstrating the bidirectional nature of these interactions. Once these cascades of interactions are initiated, they can unfold downstream in ways that can constrain developmental pathways toward stress-related pathology, and as mentioned above, can have multi-generational effects.

This need not be considered a permanent constraint, however. The very children that are highly reactive to harsh environments show remarkable plasticity and adaptability to positive, supportive environments, both behaviorally and physiologically. The combination of genetic, temperamental, and neurobiological factors work together to create a phenotype that is highly reactive to the environment, particularly the social environment, and has been implicated in stress-related disease and disorders (Boyce & Ellis, 2005). While this has been typically seen as a cost of harsh environments, it is also associated with resilience when the nature of the social environment changes, and is particularly important to consider related to adrenocortical attunement.

It is also important to understand that individual factors are inherently linked with family and broader psychosocial factors. For example, in mother–preschooler dyads, synchrony in inter-beat interval (IBI), an index of autonomic nervous system responding was examined. Family risk moderated the link between synchrony and self-regulation. In high-risk dyads, behavioral synchrony and self-regulation were higher when physiological synchrony was lower. For lower-risk dyads, higher IBI synchrony was related to both higher behavioral synchrony and higher self-regulation (Suveg, Shaffer, & Davis, 2015). Thus, examining resilience at the dyad or family level is imperative to our understanding of how early psychosocial factors influence child outcomes.

2.7 Conclusions, Implications, and Future Directions

The HPA axis is an obvious candidate for study of risk and resilience within families and other close relationships due to its role in attention to social information, memory, and regulation of gene expression (Sapolsky et al., 2000). Adrenocortical attunement has been established as a reliable biomarker that indexes shared social, emotional, and behavioral experiences. Major advantages to this approach are that collection of saliva is non-invasive, can be done in any setting, and is not subject to social desirability in the way that self-report and behavioral observations can be. In other words, it serves as an unbiased indicator of the underlying connectedness within a relationship.

While much is left to be learned about adrenocortical attunement and physiological synchrony overall within close relationships, it appears that it is a powerful predictor of developmental outcomes. Physiological and behavioral synchrony allows for the continuous exchange of information between infants and their caregivers that aids in language learning (Fletcher et al., 2005), and other aspects of cognitive and emotional development, including self-regulation (Raver, 1996). Adrenocortical attunement sets the stage for a variety of social contexts, and may be one mechanism by which attachment relationships are transferred across relationship types (e.g., parent–child attachment style associated with later romantic attachment style) (see Del Giudice, 2009). This systematic coordination of the HPA axis is best predicted by sensitivity to one's partner, in the case of children, by parental sensitivity, and appears to be most apparent during times of challenge (Ruttle, Serbin, Stack, Schwartzman, & Shirtcliff, 2011).

Our current understanding of moderating factors that serve to establish and disrupt attunement and how these fluctuations serve to impact adjustment is currently limited. We are particularly limited in our understanding of how HPA coordination within dyads and families occurs as they are going about their typical activities (outside of laboratory settings) and encountering challenges that vary in intensity and ability to coordinate responses. Furthermore, comparing attunement across groups with varying stressor types (e.g., economic stress, neighborhood violence, discrimination, domestic conflict, parental psychopathology) can illuminate moderating factors involved in the ability to establish, disrupt, and re-establish physiological coordination.

Individual, dyadic, and triadic variations in physiological functioning may act to moderate the development of behavioral, learning, and health outcomes associated with high-risk early environments (McEwen & Seeman, 1999). Importantly, alternations in physiological functioning within the family may be a vital predictor that signifies potential downstream negative developmental outcomes. This would suggest that identification of problematic physiological profiles within the family could lead to very early intervention, effectively preventing the onset of negative developmental pathways. Shifts in the coordination of physiological profiles of infants and their parents, if properly identified and placed into context, could be used as an index of the success of intervention programs.

Future studies should better delineate the relative benefits of attunement, and potentially lack of attunement in some cases. For example, as mentioned above, maternal depression has been associated with a host of negative consequences for infants and children, including altered cortisol levels. Given the relatively high frequency of maternal depression, particularly among lower socio-economic status mothers, it is important that we understand the contexts in which it may be beneficial for infants to be physiologically attuned with their caregivers, and the conditions in which withdraw from that synchrony may be advantageous. The co-regulation of physiological and behavioral responses in at-risk families specifically may serve as an important outcomes measure and window into the conscious and unconscious underpinnings of human family dynamics and human development.

Questions for Thought and Discussion

1. Much of the physiological synchrony literature focuses on the mother–infant relationship. Studies that analyze the father–child relationship often find that fathers are not directly in-sync with the child, but do demonstrate physiological synchrony with the mother, depending on level of investment in the relationship. What implications might this have on a family unit that includes a single father?
2. There is evidence that boys and girls elicit different patterns of mutual responsiveness from their caregivers. Our chapter discusses how maternal past experiences with abuse and depressive/anxiety disorders have a differential impact on the mother–infant synchrony of boys and girls. What are some possible reasons for these sex differences from a biopsychosocial standpoint?
3. What are some examples of how different family dynamics impact physiological synchrony? In what way would you predict these dynamics affect synchrony?
4. Is physiological synchrony always positive? Are there times when lack of synchrony within the family could serve as a protective factor?
5. What are some factors that protect the development of infants' stress response system in affluent families that might be lacking in economically disadvantaged families?
6. How could physiological synchrony be used to assess effectiveness of different interventions for families at risk for or experiencing adverse outcomes?
7. In our chapter, we emphasized the lack of research on fathers' influence on the family biorhythm. What impact might other family members, such as grandparents and siblings, have on infant stress response system development?

References

Beck, L. A., Pietromonaco, P. R., DeBuse, C. J., Powers, S. I., & Sayer, A. G. (2013). Spouses' attachment pairings predict neuroendocrine, behavioral, and psychological responses to marital conflict. *Journal of Personality and Social Psychology, 105*, 388–424. https://doi.org/10.1037/a0033056

Beebe, B., Alson, D., Jaffe, J., Feldstein, S., & Crown, C. (1988). Vocal congruence in mother-infant play. Journal of Psycholinguistic Research, 17, 245–259.

Belsky, J., Steinberg, L., & Draper, P. (1991). Childhood experience, interpersonal development, and reproductive strategy: An evolutionary theory of socialization. *Child Development, 62*, 647–670. https://doi.org/10.2307/1131166

Belsky, J., & Pluess, M. (2013). Beyond risk, resilience, and dysregulation: Phenotypic plasticity and human development. Development and Psychopathology 25(4pt2):1243–1261

Bigelow, A. E., MacLean, K., Proctor, J., Myatt, T., Gillis, R., & Power, M. (2010). Maternal sensitivity throughout infancy: Continuity and relation to attachment. *Infant Behavior and Development, 33*, 50–60. https://doi.org/10.1016/j.infbeh.2009.10.009

Blair, C., & Raver, C.C. (2012). Individual development and evolution: Experiential canalization of self-regulation. Developmental Psychology. 48:647–657.

Bornstein, M.H. (2009). Toward a model of culture <-> parent <-> child interactions. In A. Sameroff (Ed.), The transactional model of development: How children and contexts shape each other. Washington, DC: American Psychological Association.

Boyce, W. T., & Ellis, B. (2005). Biological sensitivity to context: I. An evolutionary-developmental theory of the origins and functions of stress reactivity. *Development and Psychopathology, 17*, 271–301. https://doi.org/10.1017/S0954579405050145

Bretherton, I., & Munholland, K. A. (2008). Internal working models in attachment relationships: Elaborating a central construct in attachment theory. In J. Cassidy & P. R. Shaver (Eds.), *Handbook of attachment: Theory, research, and clinical applications* (pp. 102–127). New York, NY: Guilford.

Byrd-Craven, J., Auer, B. J., Granger, D. A., & Massey, A. R. (2012). The father-daughter dance: The relationship between father-daughter relationship quality and daughters' stress response. *Journal of Family Psychology, 26*, 87–94. https://doi.org/10.1037/a0026588

Byrd-Craven, J., Geary, D. C., Vigil, J. M., & Hoard, M. K. (2007). One mate or two? Life history traits and reproductive variation in low-income women. *Acta Psychologica Sinica, 39*, 469–480.

Byrne, R. W., & Whiten, A. (1988). *Machiavellian intelligence*. Oxford: Oxford University Press.

Caldji, C., Tannenbaum, B., Sharma, S., Francis, D., Plotsky, P. M., & Meaney, M. J. (1998). Maternal care during infancy regulates the development of neural systems mediating the expression of fearfulness in the rat. *Proceedings of the National Academy of Sciences of the United States of America, 95*, 5335–5340. https://doi.org/10.1073/pnas.95.9.5335

Carter, A. S., Garrity-Rokous, F. E., Chazan-Cohen, R., Little, C., & Briggs-Gowan, M. J. (2001). Maternal depression and comorbidity: Predicting early parenting, attachment security, and toddler social-emotional problems and competencies. *Journal of the American Academy of Child & Adolescent Psychiatry, 40*, 18–26. https://doi.org/10.1097/00004583-200101000-00012

Cerqueira, J. J., Mailliet, F., Almeida, O. F. X., Jay, T. M., & Sousa, N. (2007). The prefrontal cortex as a key target of maladaptive response to stress. *Journal of Neuroscience, 27*, 2781–2787. https://doi.org/10.1523/JNEUROSCI.4372-06.2007

Champagne, F., & Meaney, M. J. (2001). Like mother, like daughter: Evidence for non-genomic transmission of parental behavior and stress responsivity. *Progress in Brain Research, 133*, 287–302. https://doi.org/10.1016/S0079-6123(01)33022-4

Clauss, N., Byrd-Craven, J., Kennison, S. M., & Chua, K. J. (2018). The roles of mothers' partner satisfaction and mother-infant communication in mother-infant adrenocortical attunement. *Adaptive Human Behavior & Physiology, 4*(1), 91–107.

Del Giudice, M. (2009). Sex, attachment, and the development of reproductive strategies. *Behavioral and Brian Sciences, 32*, 1–67. https://doi.org/10.1017/S0140525X09000016

Del Giudice, M. (2015). The life history model of psychopathology explains the structure of psychiatric disorders and the emergence of the p factor: A simulation study. *Clinical Psychological Science, 32*, 1–13. https://doi.org/10.1177/2167702615583628

Del Giudice, M., Ellis, B. J., & Shirtcliff, E. A. (2011). The adaptive calibration model of stress responsivity. *Neuroscience and Biobehavioral Reviews, 35*, 1562–1592. https://doi.org/10.1016/j.neubiorev.2010.11.007

Eckerman, C. O., Oehler, J. M., Hannan, T. E., & Moliter, A. (1995). The development prior to term age of very prematurely born newborns' responsiveness in an en face exchange. *Infant Behavior and Development, 18*, 283–297. https://doi.org/10.1016/0163-6383(95)90017-9

Ellis, B. J. (2004) Timing of Pubertal Maturation in Girls: An Integrated Life History Approach. Psychological Bulletin 130(6):920–958

Ellis, B. J., McFadyen-Ketchum, S., Dodge, K. A., Pettit, G. S., & Bates, J. E. (1999). Quality of early family relationships and individual differences in the timing of pubertal maturation in girls: A longitudinal test of an evolutionary model. *Journal of Personality and Social Psychology, 77*, 387–401. https://doi.org/10.1037/0022-3514.77.2.387

Ellis, B. J., Jackson, J. J., & Boyce, W. T. (2006). The stress response systems: Universality and adaptive individual differences. *Developmental Review*, 26, 175-212. https://doi.org/10.1016/j.dr.2006.02.004.

Ellis, B. J., & Boyce, T. W. (2008). Biological Sensitivity to Context. Current Directions in Psychological Science 17(3):183–187.

Essex, M. J., Klein, M. H., Eunsuk Cho, Kalin, N. H. (2002). Maternal stress beginning in infancy may sensitize children to later stress exposure: Effects on cortisol and behavior. *Biological Psychiatry, 52*(8), 776–784.

Feldman, R. (2007). Parent-infant synchrony and the construction of shared timing; physiological precursors, developmental outcomes, and risk conditions. *Journal of Child Psychology and Psychiatry, 48*, 329–354. https://doi.org/10.1111/j.1469-7610.2006.01701.x

Feldman, R. (2012). Parent-infant synchrony: A biobehavioral model of mutual influences in the formation of affiliative bonds. *Monographs of the Society for Research in Child Development, 77*, 42–51. https://doi.org/10.1111/j.1540-5834.2011.00660.x

Feldman, R., & Eidelman, A. I. (2007). Maternal postpartum behavior and the emergence of infant-mother and infant-father synchrony in preterm and full-term infants: The role of neonatal vagal tone. *Developmental Psychobiology, 49*, 290–302. https://doi.org/10.1002/dev.20220

Field, T. M. (2002). Prenatal effects of maternal depression. In S. H. Goodman & I. H. Gotlib (Eds.), *Children of depressed parents: Mechanisms of risk and implications for treatment* (pp. 59–88). Washington, DC: American Psychological Association. https://doi.org/10.1037/10449-003

Figueredo, A. J., Vasquez, G., Brumbach, B. H., Schneider, S. M. R., Sefcek, J. A., Tal, I. R., … Jacobs, W. J. (2006). Consilience and life history theory: From genes to brain to reproductive strategy. *Developmental Review, 26*, 243–275. https://doi.org/10.1016/j.dr.2006.02.002

Fletcher, K. L., Perez, A., Hooper, C., & Claussen, A. H. (2005). Responsiveness and attention during picture-book reading in 18-month-old to 24-month-old toddlers at risk. Early Child Development and Care, 175, 63–83. https://doi.org/10.1080/0300443042000230339

Flinn, M. (2006). Evolution and ontogeny of stress response to social challenges in the human child. *Developmental Review, 26*(2), 138–174

Fleming, A. S., O'Day, D. H., & Kraemer, G. W. (1999). Neurobiology of mother–infant interactions: Experience and central nervous system plasticity across development and generations. Neuroscience & Biobehavioral Reviews, 23, 673–685. https://doi.org/10.1016/S0149-7634(99)00011-1

Flinn, M. V., Nepomnaschy, P. A., Muehlenbein, M. P., & Ponzi, D. (2011). Evolutionary functions of early social modulation of hypothalamic-pituitary-adrenal axis development in humans. *Neuroscience and Biobehavioral Reviews, 35*, 1611–1629. https://doi.org/10.1016/j.neubiorev.2011.01.005

Flinn, M. V., Quinlan, R. L., Ward, C. V., & Coe, M. K. (2007). Evolution of the human family: Cooperative males, long social childhoods, smart mothers, and extended kin networks. In C. Salmon & T. Shackelford (Eds.), *Family relationships* (pp. 16–38). Oxford: Oxford University Press.

Fuchs, A., Mohler, E., Resch, F., & Kaess, M. (2016). Sex-specific differences in adrenocortical attunement in mothers with a history of childhood abuse and their 5-month-old boys and girls. *Journal of Neural Transmission, 123*, 1085–1094. https://doi.org/10.1007/s00702-016-1525-6

Francis, D.D. & Meaney, M.J. (1999). Maternal care and the development of stress responses. Current Opinion in Neurobiology, 9, 128–134.

Geary, D. C. & Bjourklund, D. F. (2000). Evolutionary Developmental Psychology. *Child Development, 71*, 57–65.

Geary, D. C., & Flinn, M. V. (2002). Sex differences in behavioral and hormonal response to social threat: Commentary on Taylor et al. (2000). *Psychological Review, 109*, 745–750. https://doi.org/10.1037/0033-295X.109.4.745

Geary, D. C. (2005). The origin of mind: Evolution of brain, cognition, and general intelligence. Washington, DC., American Psychological Association.

Geary, D. C. (2016). Evolution of sex differences in trait- and age-specific vulnerabilities. *Perspectives on Psychological Science* 855–876.

Granger, D. A., Serbin, L. A., Scwartzman, A. E., Luhoux, P., Cooperman, J., & Ikeda, S. (1998). Children's salivary cortisol, internalizing behavior problems, and family environment: Results from the Concordia Longitudinal Risk Project. *International Journal of Behavioral Development, 22*, 707–728.

Gunnar, M. R., & Donzella, B. (2002). Social regulation of cortisol levels in early human development. *Psychoneuroendocrinology, 27*(1–2), 199–220. https://doi.org/10.1016/S0306-4530(01)00045-2

Hatfield, E., Cacioppo, J. T., & Rapson, R. L. (1993). Emotional contagion. *Current Directions in Psychological Science, 2*, 96–99. https://doi.org/10.1111/1467-8721.ep10770953

Hibel, L. C., Granger, D. A., Blair, C., & Finegood, E. D. (2015). Maternal-child adrenocortical attunement in early childhood: Continuity and change. *Developmental Psychobiology, 57*, 83–95. https://doi.org/10.1002/dev.21266

Hill, K., & Kaplan, H. (1999). Life history traits in humans: Theory and empirical studies. *Annual Review of Anthropology, 28*, 397–430. https://doi.org/10.1146/annurev.anthro.28.1.397

Hofer, M. A. (1987). Early social relationships: A psychobiologist's view. *Child Development, 58*, 633–647. https://doi.org/10.2307/1130203

Hofer, M. A. (1994). Early relationships as regulators of infant physiology and behavior. Acta Paediatrica, 83, 9–18. https://doi.org/10.1111/j.1651-2227.1994.tb13260.x

Hrdy, S. B. (1999). *Mother nature: A history of mothers, infants, natural selection*. New York, NY: Pantheon.

Hrdy, S. B. (2009). *The woman that never evolved*. Cambridge, MA: Harvard University Press.

Huether, G. (1998). Stress and the adaptive self-organization of neuronal connectivity during early childhood. *International Journal of Developmental Neuroscience, 16*(3–4), 297–306. https://doi.org/10.1016/S0736-5748(98)00023-9

Iacoboni, M., Woods, R. P., Brass, M., Bekkering, H., Mazziotta, J. C., & Rizzolatti, G. (1999). Cortical mechanisms of human imitation. *Science, 286*(5449), 2526–2528. https://doi.org/10.1126/science.286.5449.2526

Kaplan, H. B., Burch, N. R., & Bloom, S. W. (1964). Physiological covariation and sociometric relationships in small peer groups. In P. H. Leiderman & D. Shapiro (Eds.), *Psychobiological approaches to social behavior* (pp. 92–109). Stanford, CA: Stanford University Press.

Keller, H., Lohaus, A., Volker, S., Elben, C., & Ball, J. (2003). Warmth and contingency and their relationship to maternal attitudes toward parenting. The Journal of Genetic Psychology, 3:275–292.

Levine, R. A. (2002). Contexts and culture in psychological research. *New Directions for Child Development* (96), 101–106. https://doi.org/10.1002/cd.46

Liu, D., Diorio, J., Tannenbaum, B., Caldji, C., Francis, D., Freedman, A., Sharma, S., Pearson, D., Plotsky, P.M., & Meaney, M.J. (1997). Maternal care, hippocampal glucocorticoid receptors, and hypothalamic-pituitary-adrenal responses to stress. Science 277:1659–1662.

Liu, S., Rovine, M. J., Cousino Klein, L., & Almeida, D. M. (2013). Synchrony of diurnal cortisol pattern in couples. *Journal of Family Psychology, 27*, 579–588. https://doi.org/10.1037/a0033735.

Lupien, S. J., McEwen, B. S., Gunnar, M. R., & Heim, C. (2009). Effects of stress throughout the lifespan on the brain, behavior and cognition. Nature Reviews Neuroscience. 10:434–445.

McEwen, B. S., & Seeman, T. (1999). Protective and damaging effects of mediators of stress: Elaborating and testing the concepts of allostasis and allostatic load. *Annals of the New York Academy of Sciences, 896*, 30–47. https://doi.org/10.1111/j.1749-6632.1999.tb08103.x

McGowan, P. O., Sasaki, A., D'Alessio, A. C., Dymov, S., Lanonte, B., Szyf, M., … Meaney, M. J. (2009). Epigenetic regulation of the glucocortiocoid receptor in human brain associates with childhood abuse. *Nature Neuroscience, 12*, 342–348. https://doi.org/10.1038/nn.2270

Meaney, M. J. (2001). Maternal care, gene expression, and the transmission of individual differences in stress reactivity across generations. *Annual Review of Neuroscience, 24*, 1161–1192. https://doi.org/10.1146/annurev.neuro.24.1.1161

Mills-Koonce, W. R., Garrett-Peters, P., Barnett, M., Granger, D. A., Blair, C., Cox, M. J., & the Family Life Project Key Investigators. (2011). Father contributions to cortisol responses in infancy and toddlerhood. *Developmental Psychology, 47*, 388–395. https://doi.org/10.1037/a0021066

Moffit, T. E., Caspi, A., & Belsky, J. (1992). Childhood experience and the onset of menarche: A test of a sociobiological model. *Child Development, 63*, 47–58. https://doi.org/10.2307/1130900

Moore, C. L., & Power, K. L. (1992). Variation in maternal care and individual differences in play, exploration, and grooming of juvenile Norway rat offspring. *Developmental Psychobiology, 25*, 165–182.

Murray, L., Kempton, C., Woolgar, M., & Hooper, R. (1993). Depressed mothers' speech to their infants and its relation to infant gender and cognitive development. *Journal of Child Psychology and Psychiatry, 34*, 1083–1101. https://doi.org/10.1111/j.1469-7610.1993.tb01775.x

Munk, A., Guyre, P.M., & Holbrook, N. J. (1984). Physiological functions of glucocorticoids in stress and their relation to pharmacological actions. *Endocrine Reviews, 5*, 25–44.

Out, D., Pieper, S., Bakermans-Kranenburg, M.J., Zeskind, P.S., & van IJzendoorn, M.H. (2010). Intended sensitive and harsh caregiving responses to infant crying: the role of cry pitch and perceived urgency in an adult twin sample. Child Abuse & Neglect 34:863–873.

Out, D. Bakermans-Kranenburg, M.J., Van Pelt, J., & Can IJzendoorn, M.H. (2012). Salivary alpa-amylase and intended harsh caregiving in response to infant crying: Evidence for physiological hyperreactivity. Child Maltreatment 17:295–305.

Papp, L. M., Pendry, P., Simon, C. D., & Adam, E. K. (2013). Spouses' cortisol associations and moderators: Testing physiological synchrony and connectedness in everyday life. *Family Process, 52*, 284–298. https://doi.org/10.1111/j.1545-5300.2012.01413.x

Pruessner, J.C., Dedovic, K., Pruessner, M., Lord, C., Buss, C., Collins, L., Dagher, A., & Lupien, S.J. (2010). Stress regulation in the central nervous system: evidence from structural and functional neuroimaging studies in human populations – 2008 Curt Richter Award Winner. Psychoneuroendocrinology 35:179–191.

Quinlan, R. J. (2003) Father absence, parental care, and female reproductive development. *Evolution and Human Behavior, 24*(6), 376–390.

Raver, C. C. (1996) Relations between social contingency in mother-child interaction and 2-year-olds' social competence. Developmental Psychology 32(5):850–859

Reid, V. M., Dunn, K., Young, R. J., Amu, J., Donovan, T., & Reissland, N. (2017). The human fetus preferentially engages with face-like visual stimuli. *Current Biology, 27*, 1825–1828. https://doi.org/10.1016/j.cub.2017.05.044

Ruttle, P. L., Serbin, L. A., Stack, D. M., Schwartzman, A. E., & Shirtcliff, E. A. (2011). Adrenocortical attunement in mother-child dyads: Importance of situational and behavioral characteristics. *Biological Psychology, 88*, 104–111. https://doi.org/10.1016/j.biopsycho.2011.06.014

Sapolsky, R. M., Romero, L. M., & Munk, A. U. (2000). How do glucocorticoids influence stress responses? Integrating permissive, suppressive, stimulatory, and preparative actions. *Endocrine Reviews, 21*, 55–89. https://doi.org/10.1210/er.21.1.55

Saxbe, D. E., Margolin, G., Shapiro, L. S., Ramos, M., Rodriguez, A., & Iturralde, E. (2014). Relative influences: Patterns of HPA axis concordance during triadic family interaction. *Health Psychology, 33*, 273–281. https://doi.org/10.1037/a0033509

Sheppard, P., Snopkowski, K., & Sear, R. (2014). Father absence and reproduction-related outcomes in Malaysia: A transitional fertility population. *Human Nature, 25*, 213–234. https://doi.org/10.1007/s12110-014-9195-2

Stearns, S. C. (1977). The evolution of life history traits: A critique of the theory and a review of the data. *Annual Review of Ecology and Systematics, 8*, 145–171. https://doi.org/10.1146/annurev.es.08.110177.001045.

Stearns, S. C. (1992). *The evolution of life histories*. Oxford: Oxford University Press.
Storey, A. E., Walsh, C. J., Quinton, R. L., & Wynne-Edwards, K. E. (2000). Hormonal correlates of paternal responsiveness in new and expectant fathers. *Evolution and Human Behavior, 21*, 79–95. https://doi.org/10.1016/S1090-5138(99)00042-2
Surbey, M. (1990). Family composition, stress, and human menarche. In F. Bercovitch & T. Zeigler (Eds.), *The socioendocrinology of primate reproduction* (pp. 71–97). New York, NY: Liss.
Suveg, C., Shaffer, A., & Davis, M. (2015). Family stress moderates relations between physiological and behavioral synchrony and child self-regulation in mother-preschooler dyads. *Developmental Psychobiology, 58*, 83–97. https://doi.org/10.1002/dev.21358
Szyf, M., Weaver, I. C. G., Champagne, F. A., Diorio, J., & Meaney, M. J. (2005). Maternal programming of steroid receptor expression and phenotype through DNA methylation in the rat. *Frontiers in Neuroendocrinology, 26*, 139–162. https://doi.org/10.1016/j.yfrne.2005.10.002
Shirtcliff, E.A., Vitacco, M.J., Graf, A.R., Gostisha, A.J. Merz, J.L., & Zahn-Waxler, C. (2009). Neurobiology of empathy and callousness: Implications for the development of antisocial behavior. Behavioral Sciences & the Law 27:173–171.
Taylor, S. E., & Gonzaga, G. C. (2006). Evolution, relationships, and health: The social shaping hypothesis. In M. Schaller, J. Simpson, & F. Kenrick (Eds.), *Evolution and Social Psychology* (pp. 211–236). Ann Arbor, MI: Sheridan.
Tester-Jones, M., O'Mahen, H., Watkins, E., & Karl, A. (2015). The impact of maternal characteristics, infant temperament and contextual factors on maternal responsiveness to infant. *Infant Behavior and Development, 40*, 1–11. https://doi.org/10.1016/j.infbeh.2015.02.014
Uchino, B. N., Uno, D., & Holt-Lunstad, J. (1999). Social support, physiological processes, and health. *Current Directions in Psychological Sciences, 8*, 145–148. https://doi.org/10.1111/1467-8721.00034
Vigil, J. M., Geary, D. C., & Byrd-Craven, J. (2006). Trade-offs in low-income women's mate preferences: Within-sex differences in reproductive strategy. *Human Nature, 17*, 319–336. https://doi.org/10.1007/s12110-006-1012-0
Waters, S. F., West, T. V., & Mendes, W. B. (2014). Stress contagion: Physiological covariation between mothers and infants. *Psychological Science, 25*, 934–942. https://doi.org/10.1177/0956797613518352
Weinberg, M. K., Beeghly, M., Olson, K. L., & Tronick, E. (2008). Effects of maternal depression and panic disorder on mother-infant interactive behavior in the face-to-face still-face paradigm. *Infant Mental Health Journal, 29*, 472–491. https://doi.org/10.1002/imhj.20193
Weinberg, M. K., Tronick, E. Z., Cohn, J. F., & Olson, K. L. (1999). Gender differences in emotional expressivity and self-regulation during early infancy. *Developmental Psychology, 35*, 175. https://doi.org/10.1037/0012-1649.35.1.175
Wynne-Edwards, K. E., & Reburn, C. J. (2000). Behavioral endocrinology of mammalian fatherhood. *Trends in Ecology & Evolution, 15*(11), 464–468. https://doi.org/10.1016/S0169-5347(00)01972-8

Chapter 3
The Heart of Conversation: Using State Space Grids to Disentangle Cardiovascular and Affect Dynamics During Couple Interaction

Clint L. Broadbent, Todd A. Spencer, Brandt C. Gardner, and Nathan Hardy

Dyadic relationships, such as couples, are dynamic systems consisting of complex interactions both within and between unique individuals. As such, couple researchers have tried to link dynamics within couple interactions to couple outcomes (Gottman & Notarius, 2000). However, researchers have suggested there is a "lack of fit" between traditional linear research methodology and studying relational systems (Granic & Hollenstein, 2003). As technology advances, novel ways to examine dyadic data in real time have emerged. One example of these advances is the use of State Space Grids (SSGs; Hollenstein, 2013) to analyze dyadic (and even triadic: Hollenstein, Allen, & Sheeber, 2016) interactions. SSGs have allowed researchers to analyze the dynamic patterns and structure that emerge in both parent–child (e.g., Lougheed, Hollenstein, & Lewis, 2016; Provenzi, Borgatti, Menozzi, & Montirosso, 2015) and couple (e.g., Gardner & Wampler, 2008; Sesemann et al., 2016) interactions using continuous data. Similarly, advances in physiological measurement have facilitated the use of physiological data in social science research. Distilling both continuous affect and continuous physiological dynamics into meaningful and useful variables may be a "next step" that yields further insight into both individual and dyadic levels of functioning. Being able to identify the synchrony between affect

C. L. Broadbent
Department of Human Development and Family Science, Oklahoma State University, Stillwater, OK, USA

Department of Teacher Education & Family Development, Southern Utah University, Cedar City, UT, USA
e-mail: clintbroadbent@suu.edu

T. A. Spencer · B. C. Gardner (✉) · N. Hardy
Department of Human Development and Family Science, Oklahoma State University, Stillwater, OK, USA
e-mail: todd.spencer@okstate.edu; brandt.gardner@okstate.edu; nathan.hardy@okstate.edu

A. W. Harrist, B. C. Gardner (eds.), *Biobehavioral Markers in Risk and Resilience Research*, Emerging Issues in Family and Individual Resilience,
https://doi.org/10.1007/978-3-030-05952-1_3

and cardiovascular activity holds potential for researchers to better understand the role of biological processes and emotional states during couple interactions.

The purpose of this chapter is to introduce an innovative strategy for measuring couple physiology and affect—known predictors of relationship outcomes and individual health. To do so, we will describe a study in which we used a novel method of data collection and analysis encompassing advanced dyadic data and within time analyses that account for continuous measures of affect and physiology. We will demonstrate the usefulness of State Space Grids to uncover trends in couples as they discuss emotionally distressing topics. The chapter will display a case example from this research and outlines steps for future research.

Social learning theory and behavioral exchange models dominated the early years of romantic relationship research—if couples communicate and manage conflict well, then they will be more satisfied in their relationships. This *behavior-perception* assumption drew researcher's attention to interactional skills (for a review see, Gottman & Notarius, 2000) as the main predictor of relationship outcomes. Levenson and Gottman's (1983) early research provided nuance to and challenged the traditional behavior-perception model as they began investigating a third construct in what Gottman would later call "the core triad of balance": *physiology* (Gottman, 1998). Although they were the first to measure it in a "love lab," it doesn't take a relationship scientist to realize that emotions run high and physiological changes take place when couples are in the "heat" of conflict. Their initial findings, however, discovered an important interplay between diffuse physiological arousal (DPA; the human stress response) and behavioral and thinking patterns during conflict—couples don't use good communication skills and don't think clearly when they are emotionally charged. Gottman saw affect (emotional states) and physiology (biological processes) so interconnected that both made up one piece of the triad and were usually measured simultaneously in their research. Gottman clarified, however, that he believed there was a difference between DPA and emotional/affective states and believed that future research would be able to clarify the different ways they connect and intersect (Gottman, 1998). Nevertheless, since this time, the majority of research have investigated these variables separately in terms of relationship outcomes.

A substantive body of research affirms the prominence of affect as an influence in both proximal and distal relationship outcomes. We understand that, even in some of the earliest observational studies of marital couples, negative affect emerged as a key indicator of relational distress (Gottman, 1979; Raush, Barry, Hertel, & Swain, 1974). Historically, research by a variety of scholars have found direct links between affect (particularly negative affect) and relationship satisfaction, to the point that some have argued that it is the most reliable predictor of current and future relationship satisfaction (e.g., Carrere & Gottman, 1999; Griffin, 1993, 2002; Mattson, Frame, & Johnson, 2011; Smith, Vivian, & O'Leary, 1990). Others have suggested that the affect expressed within couple interactions is more influential than communication skill (Johnson et al., 2005). More recently, scholars have sought to understand the moment-to-moment influence that one partner's affect can have on the other, revealing tremendous complexity in the connectedness between romantically linked individuals (Burr, Hubler, Larzelere, & Gardner, 2013; Griffin & Li, 2016).

The literature on physiological processes in romantic relationships is less robust given the complexity of the method; nevertheless, the research is growing and is quite interesting. Gottman and Levenson's longitudinal research indicated that low levels of physiological arousal during conflictual interactions were associated with higher levels of marital satisfaction (Levenson & Gottman, 1983), future marital stability (Gottman et al., 1998; Gottman & Levenson, 1992), and physical and mental health (McCarthy, King, & Levenson, 2002). Kiecolt-Glaser and colleagues studied newlyweds in their first year of marriage drawing blood to assess for adrenaline and noradrenaline employing a similar conflict discussion procedure (Kiecolt-Glaser, Bane, Glaser, & Malarkey, 2003). After following these couples for 10 years, they found that those who later divorced had significantly more adrenaline during their conflict discussion than those who stayed married. The same was true for maritally distressed couples as compared to their non-distressed counterparts. Much of the research on physiology today have linked marital interaction patterns that prompt different physiological states to individual health outcomes. For instance, three main physiological systems—cardiovascular, immune, and endocrine—are *all* adversely affected by negative and hostile conflict, and when adversely affected, predict decreases in individual health (Robles & Kiecolt-Glaser, 2003). Further, a meta-analytic analysis found that greater marital quality was related to lower cardiovascular reactivity during marital conflict and better health (Robles, Slatcher, Trombello, & McGinn, 2014).

There is limited research investigating the interrelations between affect and physiological variables. What we do know is that they are clearly correlated and both predictive of relationship satisfaction and stability (e.g., Gottman & Levenson, 1992; Levenson & Gottman, 1985), but how are we to understand the interrelations between these experiences? A common finding was that couples who were able to introduce positive emotions (e.g., affection, humor) into their conflict discussions were able to down-regulate or "soothe" physiological arousal *between* each other (e.g., Carstensen, Gottman, & Levenson, 1995; Yuan, McCarthy, Holley, & Levenson, 2010). Interestingly, greater synchrony in physiological systems has been found more in maritally satisfied than dissatisfied couples (Thomsen & Gilbert, 1998). Clearly, partner–partner exchanges of affect during conflict is part of the complexity; however, physiological arousal could also pre-set the conditions by which affect is interpreted and received. Hence, future research employing more complex methods of data collection and analysis is needed to better untangle this knot.

3.1 Theoretical Framework: Attachment Theory

Although Gottman began his research from a more data-driven position, he has since adopted *attachment* (Bowlby, 1969) as the most useful explanatory construct of his research including how physiological and affective states negatively or positively impact the long-term trajectory of romantic relationships (Gottman & Gottman, 2017). The fundamental assumption of attachment theory is that humans, beginning in infancy, emotionally attach to a primary person as a "secure base" and a "safe haven" (Bowlby, 1969). When emotional disconnection is experienced, we have three predictable patterns of responding (Ainsworth & Bell, 1970): *protest* the disconnection and demand emotional engagement (anxious response), *turn away* or disown attachment needs (avoidant response), or securely *reach out* (secure response); biologically, these moments prompt physiological distress and negative emotional/affective states. Sensing security from our attachment figure literally "soothes" our physiological arousal.

These attachment experiences do not end in childhood, but carry on into adulthood (Bowlby, 1969) where "emotional bonds" occur in important relationships across the lifespan (Waters & Cummings, 2000, p. 170). Hazan and Shaver (1987) found that attachment patterns among adults were similar to infants. Young children develop attachment "styles" of relating which are shaped by their experiences with their early attachment figure(s) based upon anxious and avoidant dimensions (Brennan, Clark, & Shaver, 1998), ranging from low (more secure) to high (less secure). These styles are found to be somewhat stable across the lifespan (e.g., Waters, Merrick, Treboux, Crowell, & Albersheim, 2000) and are predictive of how individuals approach and experience interpersonal interactions in adult romantic relationships (e.g., Brassard, Lussier, & Shaver, 2009; Creasey & Ladd, 2005; Crowell et al., 2002; Pietromonaco, Greenwood, & Barrett, 2004). Hence, adults carry an imprinted way of relating to their own romantic relationships that follow these attachment patterns.

We expect that emotionally tense conversations between partners can *feel* like threats to the attachment bond, and give rise to various physiological and negative affective responses, rooted in the attachment style by which the person orients. Sending positive messages of security is likely to soothe negative arousal during conflict discussions, but experiencing physiological arousal makes it difficult for partners to express these emotions. On the flip side, positive conversations likely trigger soothing reactions and positive affective responses, but these may be difficult to engage in after having been "triggered" by previous negative conversations. Theoretically, attachment anxiety and/or avoidance should determine, to some extent, how partners experience physiological arousal and a positive or negative affect during conversations with their partner. Overall, this is a valuable theory offering a "why" and a "how" of the physiological and affective process that occurs between partners during distress- and non-distress-related conversations.

3.2 Innovative Method: GridWare and the State Space Grid

The identification of patterns and sequences and underlying structure within what appears to be chaotic and disordered interactions is an exciting step forward in the study of individual and relational dynamics. While this has almost always been a goal of early relational researchers, we have more tools at our disposal today. One of these is GridWare (Lamey, Hollenstein, Lewis, & Granic, 2004), software designed to visually represent time-series data within a "State Space Grid." Very little research has been done using the SSG with physiological data.

GridWare allows researchers to not only visually represent continuous data, but to also derive variables from that data. We—the authors—have typically used GridWare to develop variables associated with the continuous affect reported by romantically linked partners. Immediately following a problem-solving or other type of conversation, partners engage in a video-recall procedure where they rewatch the video of their conversation and use a computer to continuously rate their affect during that conversation on a 5-point scale (high negativity = 1, neutral = 3, high positivity = 5). We then pair partners' data together and import it into GridWare, which produces a 5 × 5 SSG with one partner along the *x*-axis and the other along the *y*-axis. The data are represented by circles on the grid that vary in size by the amount of time that the couple spent in that particular state (see Fig. 3.1, for example).

GridWare allows us to create "regions" on the grid (see yellow-outlined region on Fig. 3.1) and provides us with data specific to that region. For instance, the yellow-outlined region of the sample figure is a region of "negativity"; any data point in that region indicates one or both partners reporting negative affect. We have been very interested in creating variables associated with that region, such as "negative visits" (the number of times a couple moves into the negative region) and "negative duration" (the number of seconds a couple spends in that region over the course of their conversation). Those data are then able to be used in more traditional analyses along with other variables, allowing us to capture some of the more dynamic elements of the dyad in our work.

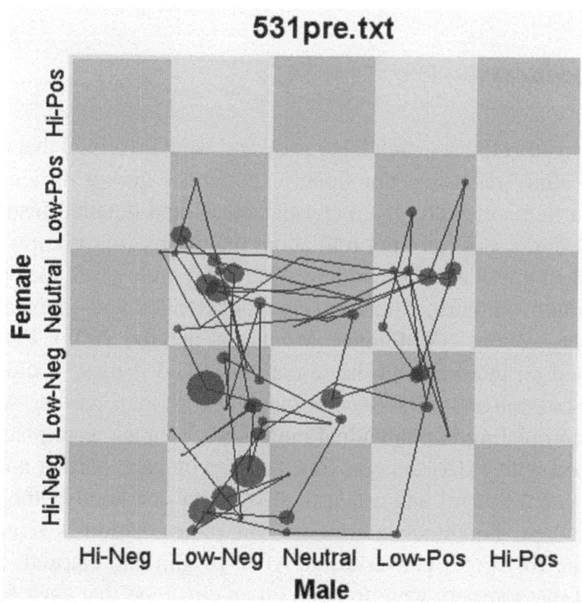

Fig. 3.1 Transitions and durations during a problem-solving discussion displayed on a State Space Grid

Our question for this particular chapter was, "Is it possible to meaningfully capture both affective and physiological elements within a single measure?" Using the SSG, can we create a within-individual measure that allows us to tease apart and still capture some of the subtleties around affect and physiology?

3.3 Methods

3.3.1 Participants

Participants were recruited using nonprobability convenience sampling procedures primarily through undergraduate classes at a southwestern university as well as local community organizations. Couples were given a gift card for their participation. Twenty-six heterosexual married couples participated in the study. The only participation criterion was that the couples needed to be married at least for 6 months. The sample was comprised of 34.6% Caucasian ($n = 18$), 7.7% Mexican-American ($n = 4$), 20.4% Asian or Pacific Islander, 7.7% American Indian or Alaska Native, and 19.2% African American ($n = 10$). The mean age of participants was 24.2 ($SD = 4.06$). The majority of participants (26.4%, $n = 11$) reported an income at or below $15,000, others reported incomes of $15,001–35,000 (22.6%, $n = 12$), $35,001–55,000 (13.2%, $n = 7$), $55,001–75,000 (11.3%, $n = 6$), more than 75,000 (9.4%, $n = 5$), and don't know/do not want to report (16.9%, $n = 9$).

3.3.2 Procedures

Participants arrived at the research laboratory and were informed that they were participating in a study regarding emotional experiences during difficult relationship discussions. Participants were given consent forms and detailed instructions about the study procedures, but were not told about the discussion prompts. Participating spouses were then interviewed separately, where they were given the prompt: "Think about a time when your partner hurt, angered, or offended you—an incident that you still have feelings about" (Waldinger, Moore, & Schulz, 2003). Participants then briefly described an incident and the researcher asked if they would be willing to engage in a discussion about the issue or incident with their partner. All participants agreed. After completing the individual interviews, couples were placed together in a room equipped with video cameras (one focused on each partner and recording to a split-screen video image) and asked to share with one another the incidents discussed during their individual interviews. This conversation is referred to as the problem-solving (or "pre") conversation. After 10 min had elapsed, a knock at the door indicated that partners were to open up an envelope that each had been given and follow the prompt on the piece of paper within. That prompt was: "Please share with your partner a time when you felt cared-for and supported by her/him, and discuss how you think such experiences affect your relationship." Couples continued this discussion, referred to as the supportive (or "post") conversation, for 7 min. Following the discussion, spouses independently reviewed the videotape of the entire conversation, and using a continuous response measure, provided a continuous rating of their affective experience during the videotaped discussion.

3.3.3 Measures

3.3.3.1 Attachment

Couples completed a survey before the couple interaction. Attachment security was assessed using the revised Experiences in Close Relationships (ECR-R; Fraley et al., 2000). The ECR-R is a 36 item self-report measure of adult attachment designed to specifically measure individual avoidance and anxiety within close relationships (Fraley et al., 2000). It has been a widely used and validated measure of adult attachment (Graham & Unterschute, 2014). Individuals in the current study were designated as either securely or insecurely attached based on their ECR-R scores that fell below the average of the sample yielding 23 securely attached individuals and 29 insecurely attached. Couples were categorized as "secure" if both members of the dyad were securely attached, and as "insecure" if one or both members of the dyad were insecurely attached.

3.3.3.2 Relationship Satisfaction

Couple relationship satisfaction was assessed using the Revised Dyadic Adjustment Scale (RDAS; Busby, Christensen, Crane, & Larson, 1995). The RDAS has been widely used to differentiate between distressed and non-distressed relationships. The RDAS is a self-report measure assessing consensus, satisfaction, and cohesion within relationships. Higher scores indicate greater stability and satisfactions, whereas lower scores indicate greater distress within the relationship.

3.3.3.3 Affect

Affect data in this study is at the couple (rather than the individual) level. Both partners reported on their affective states during the interaction to create affect scores at the couple level. Participants rated their affective experiences while watching a videotape of their couple discussions. Partners were seated at a computer displaying nine boxes on a scale. The first four boxes were labeled "negative," the middle box was labeled "neutral," and the last four boxes were labeled "positive." Participants were instructed to indicate their affective experiences during the discussion on that scale. Participants provided continuous reports of their affect as often as it changed during the discussion.

Participant's ratings of their affect were transformed into numbers on a scale from 1 (*most negative*) to 5 (*most positive*). Affect data were analyzed using GridWare, a software program designed to generate State Space Grids (SSGs) for dynamical analyses of continuous data (Lamey et al., 2004). SSGs were used to illustrate continuous affect that the partner's reported. SSGs are composed of a 5 by 5 grid to display how each partner experienced affect during the conversation. The partner's affect is then combined to see how negatively or positively the couple as a whole was during the conversation.

Affect can be measured as dynamic emotional experiences (Thompson, 1990) that include: the range of emotional experiences, changes in emotional reaction, and persistence of specific emotional response. For this study, negative affect (*negative duration and negative visits)* and affectively flexibility (*mean duration and transitions)* were the focus. Affect scores were calculated separately for the pre (problem-solving) conversation and the post (supportive) conversation. Two negativity scores were calculated: negative duration and negative visits. The negative region is indicated in Fig. 3.1 as the yellow L-shape, reflecting any time one or both partners reported feeling negatively. *Negative duration* was measured by how much time each couple spent in a negative affective state across the 17-min conversation. *Negative visits* were calculated by how many visits the couples made to a negative region during their entire 17-min conversation. This occurred when the couple moves from both partners feeling positively to one or both partners feeling negatively. In Fig. 3.1, any time the couple entered into the yellow L-shape, it would be counted as a negative visit. *Mean duration* was calculated by the average length of time that a couple spends in one affective state, whether both partners were positive, both were negative, or one was positive while the other was negative. In Fig. 3.1, the larger the circle, the more time the couple spent in that state and would be averaged to determine the mean amount of time a couple spent in each state. *Dispersion* was determined by the variety of emotional states the couple entered, specifically how many components of the 5 by 5 SSG the couple entered during their conversation. Affective *transitions per minute* were determined based on the number of times the partners changed how positively or negatively they were feeling at any one point on the 5-point scale.

Validity has been found with this measure of self-reported affect (Schuldberg & Gottlieb, 2002). This computerized, continuous self-report of affect correlates with traditional paper and pencil measures of self-reported affect, specifically the Positive and Negative Affect Scale (PANAS; Watson, Clark, & Tellegen, 1988). This measure was positively correlated with self-reports of positive affect ($r = 0.32$) and negatively correlated with self-reports of negative affect ($r = -0.30$) (Schuldberg & Gottlieb, 2002).

3.3.3.4 Cardiovascular Activity

BioPAC hardware was used to collect heart rate activity. Specifically, inter-beat interval (IBI) was selected as the cardiovascular variable due to its near-continuous nature and similarity in structure to the affect data. Inter-beat interval refers to the time between heartbeats. The smaller the interval between beats indicates an increased heart rate and greater cardiovascular arousal. Similarly, the greater the interval between heart beats indicates a slower heart rate and less cardiovascular arousal.

3.4 Analysis

Data were compiled in an excel spreadsheet and recoded and reconfigured to contain three major variables: Onset of transition, what area of affect was reported at that time (values 1–5) and what range of cardiovascular activity (IBI) was reported through the BioPAC hardware (values, 1–7). GridWare software version 1.15 for PC was used to map the results on a State Space Grid and indicate how often individuals transitioned from one of the four key zones of interest (see Fig. 3.2 for a sample grid) to another and how long they stayed in a particular zone. After analysis through GridWare, the data were entered into SPSS 25 for analysis. Due to the exploratory nature of the study and a small sample size, simple regressions were used with a *p*-value of 0.05 used as a cutoff point.

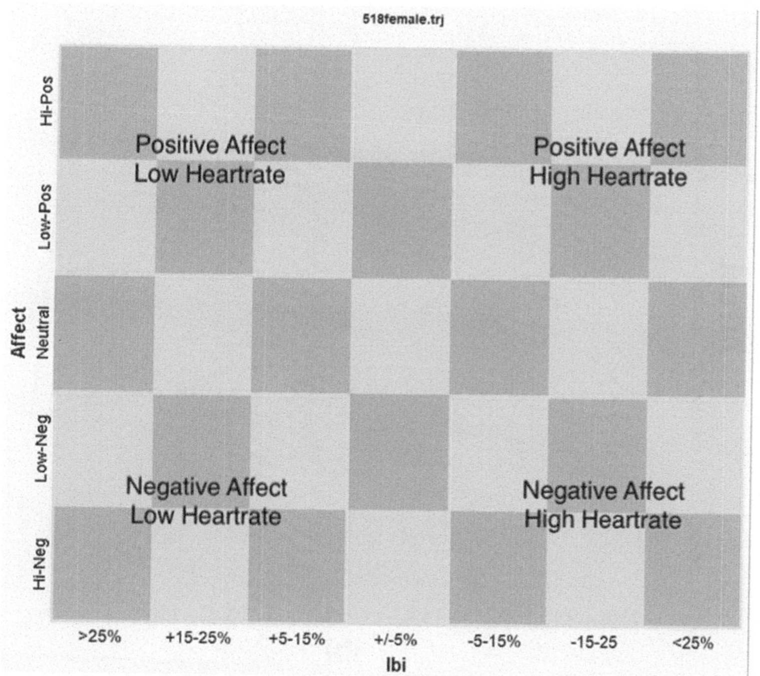

Fig. 3.2 Sample state space grid setup prior to data entry. The four primary zones of interest are highlighted and labeled.

3.5 Results

The purpose of the current study is to explore the synchrony of affect and cardiovascular activity in couples through various types of conversation. In this section, evidence for both relational and individual factors are presented (see Fig. 3.3 for a state space grid with both affect and IBI data entered).

3.5.1 *Evidence of Relational Synchrony*

When analyzing relational factors, the RDAS was significant in predicting transitions or "visits" during difficult conversations, $F(1,51) = 11.07, p < 0.05, R^2 = 0.18$. The RDAS was also able to predict where couples spend their time in the extreme zones during difficult conversations. Individuals were more likely to spend time in the positive affect high IBI zone. $F(1,51) = 6.59, p < 0.05, R^2 = 0.11$, as well as positive affect, neutral IBI area, $F(1,51) = 5.98$, $p < 0.05$, $R^2 = 0.11$. Furthermore,

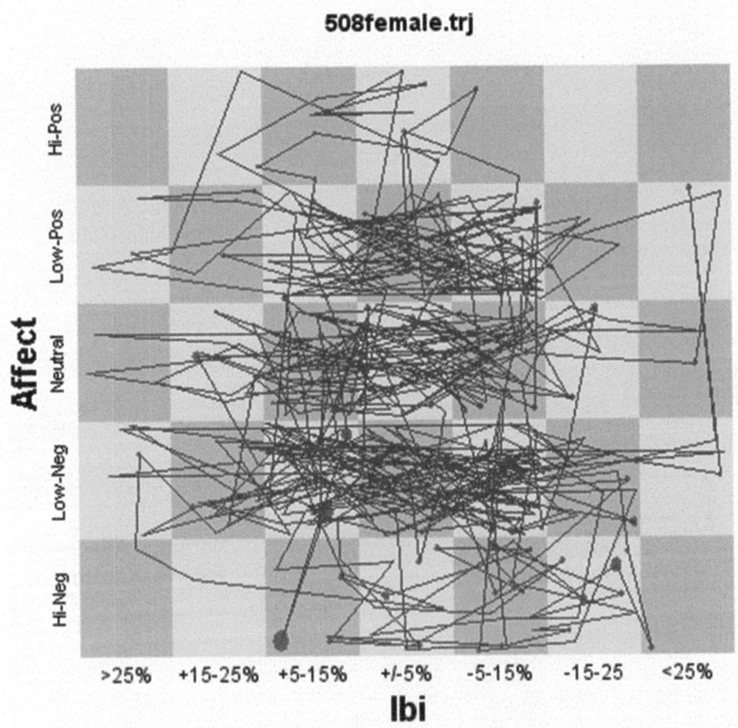

Fig. 3.3 State space grid with data from a female participant. Affect data runs along the Y-axis, and IBI data runs along the X-axis, as a percentage deviation from the individual's baseline

individuals that reported high relational satisfaction visited the negative affect, low IBI zone less during the difficult conversation, $F(1,51) = 6.56$, $p < 0.05$, $R^2 = 0.11$.

During the supportive conversations, high RDAS scores did not predict as many behaviors. In fact, the study only found that individuals tend to stay longer when visiting the positive affect, high IBI area, $F(1,51) = 4.60$, $p < 0.05$, $R^2 = 0.08$, and the positive affect, neutral IBI zones, $F(1,51) = 9.94$, $p < 0.05$, $R^2 = 0.16$, when they visit during the supportive conversation (numbers).

3.5.2 *Evidence of Effects of Individual Factors Affecting Relational Behavior*

Individual factors yielded few significant results in the study. For gender there were no significant differences in overall transitions between men and women in the supportive or difficult conversations. Visits or time spent also was not significantly different between genders. However, an analysis on visits to the positive affect, high IBI zone showed that women ($M = 24.73$, $SD = 16.06$) visit the zone significantly more than men ($M = 15.44$, $SD = 13.46$) during difficult conversations, $t(52) = 2.24$, $p < 0.05$.

Regarding attachment security, while a few variables approach significance (transitions in difficult conversations and time spent in positive affect, high IBI), there was not a difference between securely and insecurely attached individuals in the study. These insignificant findings could be a result of specific sample limitations discussed in the subsequent section.

3.6 Discussion

The purpose of the present study was to explore the potential of State Space Grids as a means to explore the synchrony between affect and cardiovascular activity among couples during a real-time interaction. Gridware was used to create a 7×5 State Space Grid that mapped participants affect and inter-beat intervals to create composite variables consisting of both affect and cardiovascular activity. Results indicate that there are potential associations between affect/cardiovascular states and relationship outcomes. For example, relationship satisfaction was a significant predictor for the number of transitions between regions during the difficult conversation. Participants who were more satisfied experienced significantly fewer transitions between affect/IBI regions than participants who reported greater relationship distress. Additionally, participants with higher relationship satisfaction were more likely to spend time in the positive affect, high IBI region than distressed couples during the difficult conversation. Such findings provide support that during difficult conversations, couples with high relationship satisfaction, report more positive affect and lower cardiovascular arousal than distressed couples.

Findings of the present study are consistent with previous research indicating that both affect and physiological responses during couple interactions are predictive of relationship satisfaction and stability (Gottman & Levenson, 1992; Levenson & Gottman, 1985). Specifically, negative affect tends to be associated with relational distress (Gottman, 1979; Raush et al., 1974) and positive affect as being one of the most reliable predictors of current and future relationship satisfaction (Carrere & Gottman, 1999; Griffin, 1993, 2002; Mattson et al., 2011; Smith et al., 1990).

Additionally, results indicate that there was no gender difference in the overall number of transitions between affect/IBI regions during the positive and supportive conversations. However, women were more likely to enter the positive affect/high IBI region than men were during the difficult conversation. Indicating that within this sample, female participants may experience more positive affect during a difficult conversation with their partner and experience less cardiovascular arousal than male participants.

The present study provides support that State Space Grids hold potential to further simultaneously examine bio-feedback and affect data within couples and individuals. Previous research has identified that dyadic relationships are dynamic systems consisting of complex interactions (Gottman & Notarius, 2002) and recent research has examined the moment-to-moment influence of one partner's affect on the other (see Burr et al., 2013; Griffin & Li, 2016). The present study contributes to the growing body of literature by using State Space Grids as a means of creating variables that simultaneously consider the real-time affect and cardiovascular activity of participants during positive and negative couple interactions. Previous research has identified that affect and physiological arousal to be associated with relationship satisfaction and stability (Gottman & Levenson, 1992; Levenson & Gottman, 1985).

3.6.1 Implications for Practice and Policy

We were able to map and monitor the interaction between affect and cardiovascular activity and its combined influence on relationship satisfaction. By further understanding the dynamic and complex process of affect and physiology during couple interactions, family scientists, educators, and therapists may be better equipped to help distressful relationships by implementing practices and interventions that target emotional and physiological regulation as part of their treatment or psycho-education. The findings of the present study indicate that individuals who report greater relationship satisfaction also report positive affect and decreased cardiovascular arousal during difficult conversations. Policy can contribute to better overall family outcomes by investing in empirically based relationship education.

Breakout Box 3.1: Focus on Practice

I will never forget my first couple's therapy case as a psychology trainee in a community mental health clinic. The tension in the room was incredibly heavy, and you could almost see the negativity bouncing back and forth between the couple like a ping pong ball. But at the same time, it was hard to know exactly what each of them was thinking or experiencing. They were talking past each other rather than to each other, and each of them was responding to something unspoken and almost invisible to me as an observer watching the match unfold. Especially as new trainee, it was overwhelming in the moment to keep up with the transactions of emotions and cognitions passing between the couple, as well as what was passing between me and each of these partners who were looking to me for help. Video recordings and live supervision became crucial tools in deciphering the patterns of emotions and cognitions in that therapy room. To be able to slow things down and more accurately recognize the points of emotional escalation and de-escalation was incredibly helpful, allowing me to more quickly and effectively anticipate hot spots in their communication. With these tools, I was better informed to help them each gain insight into the patterns driving their conflicts and to provide more targeted exercises for them to practice at home to prevent or mitigate conflict escalation. Working with couples and parent-child dyads is both a challenging and a humbling experience, namely due to the complexity of the transactions, both moment-to-moment and over longer periods of time. I have learned that the patterns of communication and behavior must first be sufficiently deciphered in order to be most effectively addressed.

—*Lucia Ciciolla,* Ph.D., Oklahoma State University

3.6.2 *Implications for Family Resilience*

This research provides support that couples in satisfying relationships may be better able to navigate difficult conversations by more frequently reporting positive affect and lower cardiovascular activation. One possible interpretation of such findings is that it may be more difficult for couples in distressed relationships to regulate their affect and physiological systems during difficult conversations. As such, distressed couples' challenges in regulating their affect and physiological systems may introduce risk for additional negative couple outcomes. Henry, Morris, and Harrist (2015) identified that a key component of family resilience is the presence of "family adaptive systems." Family adaptive systems gradually develop overtime and help regulate the day-to-day functioning of families and may moderate the potential negative effects of risk (Henry et al., 2015). One particular relevant family adaptive system for the present study is the family emotion system. Emotion regulation involves the internal and external processes individuals experience as they encounter different emotional events (Henry et al., 2015). It is likely that as couples better learn how to regulate their emotions and physiological arousal during difficult experiences with their partner that they are better able to demonstrate resilience processes in the presence of risk.

3.6.3 Future Research

Due to methodological and technological advances, there are greater avenues for investigating the role of physiology and affect in committed relationships. Granic and Hollenstein (2003) suggested that traditional linear methodology may not capture the nuances of relational systems. State Space Grids hold potential as a means to examine the association of affect and physiological measures within dyadic relationships. The present study extends the couple interaction literature by utilizing SSGs as a way of creating a composite variable consisting of both real-time affect and cardiovascular activity. Future research could use similar data collection methodologies to examine the intersection of physiological and affective experiences of couples by using SSGs and BioPac hardware. Researchers have long noted that affective and physiological responses during couple interactions are predictive of relationship satisfaction and stability (Gottman & Levenson, 1992; Levenson & Gottman, 1985). While this exploratory study focused on the association of affect/cardiovascular activity on relationship satisfaction and attachment security, future research could examine additional couple level variables beyond relationship satisfaction and attachment.

3.6.4 Limitations

While the present study makes significant contributions to understanding the synchrony of affect and cardiovascular activity it is not without limitations. Specifically, the sample consists of 26 couples. While the present study consists of dyadic data, there was insufficient power to conduct multi-level models due to sample size, as such; there are significant limitations of possible analysis without violating the assumption of independence. Additional research with a larger sample size would increase analytical options. Furthermore, there were several analyses that approached significance and a larger sample size would increase the likelihood of detecting significant relationships between variables. Additionally, the sample is fairly homogenous with a predominately Caucasian sample. As such, findings should be interpreted with caution and are limited in their generalizability.

One of the most salient limitations is the challenge associated with conducting analysis comparing the difficult conversation with the supportive conversation. Participants discussed about a time they felt hurt by their partner for 7 min before given the prompt to discuss a time they felt cared-for by their partner for 5 min.

Given the discrepancy in time spent in each condition, it is difficult to compare the number transitions between affect/IBI regions or mean duration in a particular region between the difficult conversation and positive conversation. As such, the present study examined the difficult conversation and positive conversation separately from each other. Additional research using equitable time spent in both difficult and positive conversations are required to discern differences between the difficult and positive conversation.

Questions for Thought and Discussion

1. The present study found that relationship distress was associated with greater movement between affect/cardiovascular regions during the difficult conversation. Why might we not see the same pattern during the positive conversation?
2. What are the clinical implications of affect and physiological synchrony?
3. Previous dyadic researchers have identified that there is "lack of fit" between traditional linear research methodology and studying relational systems (Granic & Hollenstein, 2003). What are the unique challenges associated with studying couples?
4. What are the benefits of studying "real-time" couple interactions?
5. The present study used State Space Grids as a within-individual measure to capture both affect and cardiovascular activity. What are other potential uses of State Space Grids?
6. Discuss the unique methodological procedures utilized in the present study. What are their strengths and limitations?

References

Ainsworth, M. D. S., & Bell, S. M. (1970). Attachment, exploration, and separation: Illustrated by the behavior of one-year-olds in a strange situation. *Child Development, 41*, 49–67. https://doi.org/10.2307/1127388

Bowlby, J. M. (1969). *Attachment and loss* (Attachment) (Vol. 1). New York, NY: Basic Books.

Brassard, A., Lussier, Y., & Shaver, P. R. (2009). Attachment, perceived conflict, and couple satisfaction: Test of a mediational dyadic model. *Family Relations, 58*, 634–646. https://doi.org/10.1111/j.1741-3729.2009.00580.x

Burr, B. K., Hubler, D. S., Larzelere, R. E., & Gardner, B. C. (2013). Applying the actor-partner interdependence model to micro-level analyses of marital partner affect during couple conversations: An exploratory investigation. *Marriage & Family Review, 49*, 284–308. https://doi.org/10.1080/01494929.2012.762446

Busby, D. M., Christensen, C., Crane, D. R., & Larson, J. H. (1995). A revision of the dyadic adjustment scale for use with distressed and nondistressed couples: Construct hierarchy and multidimensional scales. *Journal of Marital and Family Therapy, 21*, 289–308. https://doi.org/10.1111/j.1752-0606.1995.tb00163.x

Brennan, K. A., Clark, C. L., Shaver, P. R. (1998). Self-report measurement of adult attachment: An integrative overview. In J. A. Simpson & W. S. Rholes (Eds.), *Attachment theory and close relationships* (pp. 46–76). New York, NY: Guilford Press.

Carrere, S., & Gottman, J. M. (1999). Predicting divorce among newlyweds from the first three minutes of a marital conflict discussion. *Family Process, 38*, 293–301. https://doi.org/10.1111/j.1545-5300.1999.00293.x

Carstensen, L. L., Gottman, J. M., & Levenson, R. W. (1995). Emotional behavior in long-term marriage. *Psychology and Aging, 10*, 140–149. https://doi.org/10.1037/0882-7974.10.1.140

Creasey, G., & Ladd, A. (2005). Generalized and specific attachment representations: Unique and interactive roles in predicting conflict behaviors in close relationships. *Personality and Social Psychology Bulletin, 31*(8), 1026–1038. https://doi.org/10.1177/0146167204274096

Crowell, J. A., Treboux, D., Gao, Y., Fyffe, C., Pan, H., & Waters, E. (2002). Assessing secure base behavior in adulthood: Development of a measure, links to adult attachment representations and relations to couples' communication and reports of relationships. *Developmental Psychology, 38*, 679–693. https://doi.org/10.1037/0012-1649.38.5.679

Fraley, R. C., Waller, N. G., Brennan, K. A. (2000). An item response theory analysis of self-report measures of adult attachment. *Journal of Personality and Social Psychology, 78*(2), 350–365.

Gardner, B. C., & Wampler, K. S. (2008). Uncovering dynamical properties in the emotional system of married couples. *Contemporary Family Therapy, 30*, 111–126. https://doi.org/10.1007/210591-008-9056-4

Gottman, J. M. (1979). Detecting cyclicity in social interaction. *Psychological Bulletin, 86*, 338–348. https://doi.org/10.1037/0033-2909.86.2.338

Gottman, J. M., & Notarius, C. I. (2000). Decade review: Observing marital interaction. *Journal of Marriage and Family, 62*, 927–947. https://doi.org/10.1111/j.1741-3737.2000.00927.x

Gottman, J. M., Levenson, R. W. (1992). Marital processes predictive of later dissolution: Behavior, physiology, and health. *Journal of Personality and Social Psychology, 63*(2), 221–233.

Gottman, J. M. (1998). Psychology and the study of marital processes. *Annual Review of Psychology, 49*(1), 169–197.

Gottman, J., Gottman, J. (2017). The natural principles of love. *Journal of Family Theory Review, 9*(1), 7–26.

Gottman, J. M., Notarius, C. I. (2002). Marital research in the 20th century and a research agenda for the 21st century. *Family Process, 41*(2), 159–197.

Gottman, J. M., Coan, J., Carrere, S., Swanson, C. (1998). Predicting marital happiness and stability from newlywed interactions. *Journal of Marriage and the Family, 60*(1), 5.

Graham, J. M., Unterschute, M. S. (2014). A reliability generalization meta-analysis of self-report measures of adult attachment. *Journal of Personality Assessment, 97*(1), 31–41.

Granic, I., & Hollenstein, T. (2003). Dynamic systems methods for models of developmental psychopathology. *Development and Psychopathology, 15*(03), 641–669

Griffin, W. A. (1993). Transitions from negative affect during marital interaction: Husband and wife differences. *Journal of Family Psychology, 6*, 230–244. https://doi.org/10.1037/0893-3200.6.3.230

Griffin, W. A. (2002). Affect pattern recognition: Using discrete hidden Markov models to discriminate distressed from nondistressed couples. *Marriage & Family Review, 34*, 139–163.

Griffin, W. A., & Li, X. (2016). Using Bayesian nonparametric hidden semi-Markov models to disentangle affect processes during marital interaction. *PLoS One, 11*, e0155706. https://doi.org/10.1371/journal.pone.0155706

Henry, C. S., Morris, A. S., & Harrist, A. W. (2015). Family resilience: Moving into the third wave. *Family Relations, 64*, 22–43. https://doi.org/10.1111/fare.12106

Hollenstein, T. (2013). *State space grids: Depicting dynamics across development*. New York, NY: Springer.

Hollenstein, T., Allen, N. B., & Sheeber, L. (2016). Affective patterns in triadic family interactions: Associations with adolescent depression. *Development and Psychopathology, 28*, 85–96. https://doi.org/10.1017/S0954579415000309

Hazan, C., Shaver, P. (1987). Romantic love conceptualized as an attachment process. *Journal of Personality and Social Psychology, 52*(3), 511–524.

Johnson, M. D., Cohan, C. L., Davila, J., Lawrence, E., Rogge, R. D., Karney, B. R., … Bradbury, T. N. (2005). Problem-solving skills and affective expressions as predictors of change in marital satisfaction. *Journal of Consulting and Clinical Psychology, 73*, 15–27. https://doi.org/10.1037/0022-006X.73.1.15

Kiecolt-Glaser, J. K., Bane, C., Glaser, R., & Malarkey, W. B. (2003). Love, marriage, and divorce: Newlyweds' stress hormones foreshadow relationship changes. *Journal of Consulting and Clinical Psychology, 71*, 176–188. https://doi.org/10.1037/0022-006X.71.1.176

Lamey, A., Hollenstein, T., Lewis, M. D., & Granic, I. (2004). GridWare (Version 1.1). [Computer software]. Retrieved from http://statespacegrids.org

Levenson, R. W., & Gottman, J. M. (1983). Marital interaction: Physiological linkage and affective exchange. *Journal of Personality and Social Psychology, 45*(3), 587–597. https://doi.org/10.1037/0022-3514.45.3.587

Levenson, R. W., & Gottman, J. M. (1985). Physiological and affective predictors of change in relationship satisfaction. *Journal of Personality and Social Psychology, 49*, 85–94. https://doi.org/10.1037/0022-3514.49.1.85

Lougheed, J., Hollenstein, T., & Lewis, M. D. (2016). Maternal regulation of daughters' emotion during conflicts from early to mid-adolescence. *Journal of Research on Adolescence, 26*, 610–616. https://doi.org/10.1111/jora.12211

Mattson, R. E., Frame, L. E., & Johnson, M. D. (2011). Premarital affect as a predictor of postnuptial marital satisfaction. *Personal Relationships, 18*, 532–546. https://doi.org/10.1111/j.1475-6811.2010.01315.x

McCarthy, M. E., King, A. R., & Levenson, R. W. (2002, October). *Reactivity and resiliency in older adults: A twelve-year follow up*. Poster presented at the annual meeting of the Society for Psychophysiological Research, Washington, DC

Pietromonaco, P. R., Greenwood, D., & Barrett, L. F. (2004). Conflict in adult close relationships: An attachment perspective. In W. S. Rholes & J. A. Simpson (Eds.), *Adult attachment: Theory, research, and clinical implications* (pp. 267–299). New York, NY: Guilford.

Provenzi, L., Borgatti, R., Menozzi, G., & Montirosso, R. (2015). A dynamic system analysis of dyadic flexibility and stability across the face-to-face still-face procedure: Application of the state space grid. *Infant Behavior and Development, 38*, 1–10. https://doi.org/10.1016/j.infbeh.2014.10.001

Raush, H. L., Barry, W. A., Hertel, R. K., & Swain, M. A. (1974). *Communication conflict and marriage*. Oxford, UK: Jossey-Bass.

Robles, T. F., & Kiecolt-Glaser, J. K. (2003). The physiology of marriage: Pathways to health. *Physiology & Behavior, 79*, 409–416. https://doi.org/10.1016/S0031-9384(03)00160-4

Robles, T. F., Slatcher, R. B., Trombello, J. M., & McGinn, M. M. (2014). Marital quality and health: A meta-analytic review. *Psychological Bulletin, 140*, 140–187. https://doi.org/10.1037/a0031859

Schuldberg, D., & Gottlieb, J. (2002). Dynamics and correlates of microscopic changes in affect. *Nonlinear Dynamics, Psychology, and Life Sciences, 6*(3), 231–257.

Smith, D. A., Vivian, D., & O'Leary, K. D. (1990). Longitudinal prediction of marital discord from premarital expressions of affect. *Journal of Consulting and Clinical Psychology, 58*, 790–798. https://doi.org/10.1037/0022-006X.58.6.790

Sesemann, E. M., Kruse, J., Gardner, B. C., Broadbent, C. L., & Spencer, T. A. (2016). Observed attachment and self-report affect within romantic relationships. *Journal of Couple and Relationship Therapy, 16*(2), 102–121.

Thompson, R. A. (1990). Emotion and self-regulation. In Nebraska Symposium on Motivation. 1988: Socioemotional development. Current theory and research in motivation (Vol. 36, pp. 367–467). Lincoln, NE: University of Nebraska Press.

Thomsen, D. G., & Gilbert, D. G. (1998). Factors characterizing marital conflict states and traits: Physiological, affective, behavioral, and neurotic variable contributions to marital conflict and satisfaction. *Personality and Individual Differences, 25*, 833–855. https://doi.org/10.1016/S0191-8869(98)00064-6

Waters, E., Merrick, S., Treboux, D., Crowell, J., & Albersheim, L. (2000). Attachment security in infancy and early adulthood: A 20-year longitudinal study. *Child Development, 71*, 684–689. https://doi.org/10.1111/1467-8624.00176

Waters, E., Cummings, E. M. (2000). A secure base from which to explore close relationships. *Child Development, 71*(1), 164–172.

Waldinger, R. J., Moore, C., Schulz, M. S. (2003). *Child abuse and adult attachment: Links with emotion during video recall of couple interactions. Workshop presented at the annual conference of the Society for Research in Child Development.* FL: Tampa.

Watson, D., Clark, L. A., Tellegen, A. (1988). Development and validation of brief measures of positive and negative affect: The PANAS scales. *Journal of Personality and Social Psychology, 54*(6), 1063–1070.

Yuan, J. W., McCarthy, M., Holley, S. R., & Levenson, R. W. (2010). Physiological down-regulation and positive emotion in marital interaction. *Emotion, 10*, 467–474. https://doi.org/10.1037/a0018699

Chapter 4
Intergenerational Transmission of Poverty: How Low Socioeconomic Status Impacts the Neurobiology of Two Generations

Rebekah Tribble and Pilyoung Kim

Adverse physical health, cognitive, school achievement, emotional and behavioral outcomes have been documented in children living in poverty. These adverse health outcomes are thought to arise from the cumulative stress exposure that often occurs in children living in poverty. Children from lower SES exhibited altered brain development and elevated allostatic load compared to individuals from higher SES (Dohrenwend, 1973), thus individuals from lower SES likely have greater vulnerability to stress and disease.

Poverty can be a stressor for not only children but their parents. Exposure to chronic and severe stressors associated with socioeconomic disadvantage interferes with normative psychological and neurobiological changes that support motherhood during the early postpartum period (Kim & Bianco, 2014; Kim, Capistrano, & Congleton, 2016). Greater exposure to chronic and daily stressors experienced by low-income women place them at increased risk for developing depressive symptoms (Kim & Bianco, 2014). Thus the mental health of parents, which can have a critical impact on infant health and development, is negatively impacted by poverty.

Given the role of poverty in two generations—parents and children, we suggest a two-generational approach to intervention is critical to enhance resilience in families. Involving children in programs which teach them a flexible set of positive coping methods and an achievement orientation in and outside of school may help negate the negative impacts of poverty. Additionally, teaching parents coping strategies they can use to better their own well-being is imperative, specifically for their ability to effectively parent their children. Self-regulation and emotional reactivity between children and their parents seem to be related, likely bidirectional in nature (Belsky, Pasco Fearon, & Bell, 2007), with the degree of conflict during interactions related to both children's and parent's self-regulation skills (Eisenberg, 2008).

R. Tribble · P. Kim (✉)
Department of Psychology, University of Denver, Denver, CO, USA
e-mail: Rebekah.Tribble@du.edu; Pilyoung.Kim@du.edu

A. W. Harrist, B. C. Gardner (eds.), *Biobehavioral Markers in Risk and Resilience Research*, Emerging Issues in Family and Individual Resilience,
https://doi.org/10.1007/978-3-030-05952-1_4

Poverty is a public health concern and crisis. According to the US Census Bureau, 43.1 million people were living in poverty in 2015. Rates of poverty are higher among minorities (Massey & Eggers, 1990) and low socioeconomic status is related to many morbidities making those who live in poverty at greater risk for mortality due to obesity, high blood pressure, diabetes, cancer, and psychopathologies of mood such as depression (Shammas, 2011; Sobal & Stunkard, 1989; Stepnowsky, Nelesen, DeJardin, & Dimsdale, 2004; Wang & Zhang, 2006; Wilson, Kliewer, Plybon, & Sica, 2000). In the United States, poverty is defined as an income-to-needs ratio below one, calculated using total income and number of household members. In addition to poverty, many researchers interested in studying the impacts of income and social status measures use socioeconomic status (SES) to define their sample. This measure is often a combination of education, income, and occupation. Additionally, low SES is correlated with poverty. Thus, this review will include a discussion of articles that relate to both low socioeconomic status and poverty.

4.1 Poverty and Children

According to the US Census Bureau, in 2015 19.7% of children were living in poverty, which is often related to a less enriched environment. The environment of poverty is stressful for children, as many stressors such as exposure to violence, pollutants, crime, traffic, low housing quality, and unstable housing (Bradley & Corwyn, 2002; Evans, 2004) accompany living in low socioeconomic status areas. One mechanism in which poverty impacts children is through cumulative risk exposure (Evans & Kim, 2007), which is measured using multiple physical and social risk factors such as crowding, noise, family turmoil, and exposure to violence. Multiple stressors overwhelm the body, compromising its ability to efficiently handle environmental demands.

The outcomes for children living in poverty are typically a lot less favorable than those of their higher economic status peers. Studies of children's early cognitive and physical development suggest that family income in the first 5 years of life is a powerful correlate of developmental outcomes in early and middle childhood (Duncan, Brooks-Gunn, & Klebanov, 1994; Miller & Korenman, 1994; Smith, Brooks-Gunn, & Klebanov, 1997). For cognitive development, family income has been shown to be correlated with age-5 IQ, with lower IQs being associated with lower income (Duncan et al., 1994). For behavioral development, low-income children are at increased risk for developing behavioral problems (Chapman, Dube, & Anda, 2007; van Oort, van der Ende, Wadsworth, Verhulst, & Achenbach, 2011). Higher externalizing behavior scores are related to a higher proportion of low-income neighbors (Duncan et al., 1994). Prolonged poverty also significantly predicts children's internalizing symptoms (Chen, Matthews, & Boyce, 2002; Gilman, Kawachi, Fitzmaurice, & Buka, 2002; McLeod & Shanahan, 1993). Furthermore, children living in poverty are more likely to be of low birth weight (Paneth, 1995), have developmental delays, learning disabilities (Farah et al., 2006), and physical illnesses (Kollerud, Blaasaas, & Claussen, 2015; Malcolm, MacKay, Shepherd, & Weaver, 2004; Ogden, Lamb, Carroll, & Flegal, 2010; Wang & Zhang, 2006).

An adverse impact of childhood poverty across several developmental outcomes exists. As a mechanism, researchers have highlighted the impact of poverty and related chronic stress on brain development and physiological stress regulation systems. Childhood is a sensitive period for neurobiological development, thus the neurobiological system is more vulnerable to poverty exposure and severe stress during these years with a long-term impact.

4.1.1 Impact of Poverty on Childhood Brain

Poverty may impact brain development in childhood. The long-lasting impact of poverty in the brain has been highlighted as a neurobiological mechanism by which poverty influences cognitive, emotional, and physical development (Ganzel, Kim, Gilmore, Tottenham, & Temple, 2013; Gianaros et al., 2008).

Research has displayed poverty and low SES as having a negative impact on the developing brain by impacting neural structural development. Brain scans done on children aged 5–17 years, revealed individual variation in the size of discrete brain regions that are critical for language, memory, and socioemotional processing based on socioeconomic status (Noble, Houston, Kan, & Sowell, 2012). In this study, income-to-needs ratio was correlated with child hippocampal volume and number of years of parent education was negatively correlated with amygdala volume. Additionally, the left superior temporal gyrus and left inferior frontal gyrus, two language supporting regions, were positively correlated with parental education. This may explain why differences in achievement between low and high socioeconomic status children exist. In a later study, a quadratic relationship between family income and cortical surface area in many overlapping neural regions was observed such that lower income families were more affected by even very small income changes compared to children of higher income families (Noble et al., 2015). Lower neurocognitive abilities were observed in the low income children, explained by differences in cortical surface area. Additionally, a recent study looking at academic achievement between higher and lower income eighth grade students discovered cortical gray-matter volume and cortical thickness was greater in students from higher income when compared to lower income backgrounds (Mackey et al., 2015). Higher income was also associated with better test performance on a state wide exam. This study exemplifies the academic achievement gap that currently exists between children with low versus high-income backgrounds. Hair and colleagues found that children 1.5 times the general poverty line had gray mater volumes 3–4 percentage points below the developmental norm. This increased to 8–10 percentage points below the norm when income was beneath the federal poverty level. Children from low-income households also scored 4–7 points lower on standardized tests (Hair, Hanson, Wolfe, & Pollak, 2015).

Poverty can have a major impact on whole brain functioning even at a young age. In a longitudinal study, preschoolers aged 3–5 where followed up with annual behavioral assessments and scanned at school age (7–12 years old). Lower income was associated with reduced connectivity between the hippocampus and amygdala. Additionally, lower INR predicted greater negative mood and depression at school age (Barch et al., 2016). Functional connectivity of brain areas critical for emotion regulation are influenced by poverty, and these changes in connectivity are a mediating factor by which poverty is associated with subsequent negative emotional and mental health outcomes. In adolescents, increased amygdala responses to angry faces were associated with low socioeconomic status (Muscatell et al., 2012). This heightened activation to negative stimuli displays how low SES adolescents may perceive a social situation differently, such as heightened vigilance to social threats, than there middle and high socioeconomic peers.

Even in the first year of life the impacts of socioeconomic status on brain functionality have been observed, with higher income and maternal education associated with better network maturation in infants as young as 6 months of age (Gao et al., 2015). This age serves as a developmental milestone as infants learn to sit up and are more able to explore their environment in an enriching manner. Adverse long-term impacts on child development may occur from delayed development in these brain networks due to exposure to low SES at a very young age. In 6–9-month-old infants, low income and lower maternal occupation were associated with lower frontal gamma power (Tomalski et al., 2013). Resting gamma activity has been linked to differences in language and cognitive skills in toddlers (Benasich, Gou, Choudhury, & Harris, 2008), thus risk for poor language outcomes, more prevalent in low SES children, may be associated with reduced frontal gamma activity.

Children living in low SES families aged 7–12 years showed reduced activation compared to their high SES peers during a target detection task designed to assess cognitive flexibility and working memory both related to lateral prefrontal cortex activity (Kishiyama, Boyce, Jimenez, Perry, & Knight, 2009). Executive functioning and family SES was explored in 8–12 year olds revealing that low SES children exhibited more activation in the right middle frontal gyrus and with increased activation greater accuracy, compared to high SES children during a dimensional change card sorting task (Sheridan, Sarsour, Jutte, D'Esposito, & Boyce, 2012). This increased activation is likely due to the low SES children spending more time understanding the role associations during the task leading to more recruitment in this brain region in order to perform at the same level as their high SES peers.

4.1.2 Impacts of Poverty on Childhood Physiological Stress Regulation

Living under conditions of poverty and/or low SES may have physiological impacts on children even down to their DNA. Telomeres, a region of repetitive nucleotide sequences at the end of each chromosome that protects them from deterioration, have been shown to shorten with age and can serve as a biological clock to determine the lifespan of a cell or organism (Shammas, 2011). Additionally, telomere length has been suggested as a potential biomarker for lifetime exposure to stress. Accelerated telomere shortening is associated with many lifestyle factors such as obesity, smoking, poor diet, and lack of exercise. In a study of 9-year-old African American boys, low income, low maternal education, unstable family structure, and harsh parenting were all associated with shorter telomeres (Mitchell et al., 2014). Family violence and instability, which occurs in households of all income brackets but is more likely to occur in households living in poverty, especially severe violence (Gelles, 1992; McCloskey, Figueredo, & Koss, 1995) is associated with telomere length. In children aged 5–15 years, those who experienced the highest adversity had significantly shorter buccal telomere length. Additionally those who were exposed to violence, family disruption, or family instability all had shorter telomeres than children unexposed to those stressors (Drury et al., 2014).

Stressors activate cortisol, a hormone secreted by the HPA axis, which is often dysregulated in children and adolescents exposed to poverty and low SES. Hyperactivity of this stress response system is typically associated with elevated baseline levels also characteristic of children (Essex, Klein, Cho, & Kalin, 2002; Evans & English, 2002; Flinn & England, 1997; Gustafsson, Gustafsson, & Nelson, 2006; Lupien, King, Meaney, & McEwen, 2000, 2001), and adolescents (Evans & Kim, 2007) living in low SES. Cumulative exposure to poverty, measured by the number of time points when the child was 7–48 months old that caregivers reported living in poverty, results in a less steep trajectory across the day of cortisol secretion, a characteristic of HPA dysregulation (Blair, Berry, Mills-Koonce, & Granger, 2013). A cross-sectional study of children aged 4–18 years of age resulted in lower neighborhood SES being associated with higher hair cortisol and hair cortisone with higher hair cortisol correlated with lower maternal education and hair cortisone with lower paternal education (Vliegenthart et al., 2016). This chronic stress related to higher hair cortisol may mediate the association between SES and adverse outcomes for children living in low SES and poverty.

Children exposed to poverty and low SES exhibit elevated inflammatory responses. The immune system launches an inflammatory response when the body is injured or infected resulting in white blood cells collecting at the distressed site (G. E. Miller & Chen, 2013). This inflammatory response is essential for our survival, however if it becomes persistent the response can lead to various diseases. Asthma is a chronic disease that manifests from elevated inflammatory responses in our airways. Children aged 9–18 years diagnosed with asthma from lower SES had heightened production of IL-5, IL-3, and higher eosinophil counts when compared to children with asthma from higher SES (Chen et al., 2006). Children 8–10 years of age who experienced persistent low SES since birth had elevated immune responses with 70% higher IL-6 responses compared to middle SES children (Azad et al., 2012).

Last, dysregulation of multiple physiological systems at once can be thought of as allostatic load. Low SES and poverty is associated with higher allostatic load (Evans, Chen, Miller, & Seeman, 2012; Miller & Chen, 2013; Seeman, Epel, Gruenewald, Karlamangla, & McEwen, 2010). A study of rural 8–10-year-old children collected overnight urine samples to measure cumulative output of epinephrine. This study found higher levels of epinephrine among children whose family incomes were below the poverty line versus in the middle-class range (Evans & English, 2002). A portion of this sample was followed over the next 3–4 years and cumulative adversity, defined as a composite of poverty, family turmoil, and other factors, was associated with accelerated allostatic load overtime. Children who had more cumulative risk at study entry showed larger increases in allostatic load scores over the follow-up (Evans & Kim, 2007). Similarly, a study looking at cardiovascular risk in adolescents collected data from high school students and observed that students with parents reporting lower education had higher allostatic load (e.g., higher insulin, greater insulin resistance, higher LDL cholesterol) displaying wear and tear to multiple physiological systems (Goodman, McEwen, Huang, Dolan, & Adler, 2005). African American youth who lived in neighborhoods in which poverty levels increased from ages 11 to 19 had the highest levels of allostatic load (Brody, Lei, Chen, & Miller, 2014). Allostatic load in adolescents 12–19 years old was assessed using data from the United States National Health and Nutrition Exam Survey, discovering higher allostatic load in lower SES adolescents (Rainisch & Upchurch, 2013). Low SES and poverty alter stress regulatory systems, which may impact a child's ability to cope with stress, furthering their risk for illness and disease.

4.2 Poverty and Parenting

Parents may be impacted by poverty, which in turn impacts their children. Parents of children living in low SES are more likely to have lower parenting quality, as observed in video-taped mother–child interactions, rated as having less sensitivity, less positive regard and less supportive presence and quality of assistance on a puzzle task (Lugo-Gil & Tamis-LeMonda, 2008). Parents face the challenge of raising children with few resources and the accompanying risks of poverty, resulting in much added stress that impacts parental well-being (Howard, 2000; Magnuson & Duncan, 2002). Difficulties in adjustment to parenthood may also lead to a higher risk for mood disorders among parents. Mood disorders are common in mothers living in poverty, specifically in this population postpartum depression occurs at a higher rate (Walker, Timmerman, Kim, & Sterling, 2002). Clearly, the environment that parents are surrounded by may greatly impact their ability to parent.

Poverty is potentially a very important influencer on parenting (Wilson, 1987). Studies have shown that when parents live among neighbors who have limited incomes or are unemployed they often display less warmth and higher levels of discipline with their children (Simons, Johnson, Conger, & Lorenz, 1997). Additionally, parenting styles involving more harsh discipline and/or inconsistent discipline have been related to poverty (Earls, McGuire, & Shay, 1994; Furstenberg et al., 1993; Jarrett, 1997). Children with more behavior problems often have parents who display less warmth, report lower levels of appropriate, consistent discipline and have higher levels of harsh interactions (Pinderhughes, Nix, Foster, & Jones, 2001). Harsh parenting impacts the strength of the family unit and parent–child relations in a negative manner.

Many mothers living in poverty experience postpartum depression at a higher rate (Walker et al., 2002). Greater exposure to chronic and daily stressors experienced by low-income women place them at increased risk for developing depressive symptoms (Kim & Bianco, 2014). Depression impacts not only the mothers' mental health but also her ability to effectively parent her child, the relationship she builds with her child and her child's long-term development. Severity of postpartum depression has been associated with poor infant cognitive functioning (Murray, 1992). Mothers living in poverty are less likely to engage in interactive play and learning which may detrimentally impact a child's development. They are also less likely to provide their children with stimulating books (Bus, Van Ijzendoorn, & Pellegrini, 1995; Field, 2010). Thus, the mental health of parents may also have a critical impact on infant health and development as it impacts their parenting.

4.2.1 Impacts of Poverty on Neurobiological Mechanisms of Parenting

Parenting plays a large role in the development of a child. There are specific neurobiological mechanisms in place that help assist parents with growing a bond with their children. For example, mothers exhibit structural growth in multiple brain regions during the first few months postpartum (Kim et al., 2010). During the first few months, postpartum increased gray-matter volumes in large regions of the prefrontal cortex, parietal lobe, and midbrain were observed. These plastic changes in the brain help support parental motivation, properly equipping mothers to take on the daunting task of raising a child. Furthermore, a mother's positive thoughts of her baby at the first month postpartum predicted gray-matter volume increase from the first month to 3–4 months postpartum. This illustrates a biological change that may help mothers when responding to their infants especially under early postpartum circumstances that may be overwhelming and stressful in nature.

New mothers living in poverty have higher levels of maternal distress compared to their middle-income counterparts, a main reason for more negative transitions to motherhood (Goyal, Gay, & Lee, 2010). Specifically, being exposed to chronic and severe stressors that are associated with socioeconomic disadvantage may prevent normative psychological and neurobiological changes that support motherhood during the early postpartum period (Kim & Bianco, 2014). Neuroimaging studies show increased activity in response to infant cues in neural regions including the midbrain, medial, middle, and lateral prefrontal cortex; and sensorimotor and auditory cortex (Barrett & Fleming, 2011; Swain et al., 2014). In order to adapt to motherhood, new mothers exhibit enhanced neural sensitivity to infant cues, including infant cry sounds during the early postpartum period (Kim et al., 2016). Mothers living in socioeconomic disadvantage are more likely to exhibit difficulties in adjusting to motherhood. This is supported by the family stress model which states that living in a low-income environment may lead to higher levels of psychological distress among mothers (Conger, Ge, Elder, Lorenz, & Simons, 1994). This negative impact on mothers in turn increases risks for negative mother–child relationships (Newland, Crnic, Cox, & Mills-Koonce, 2013). Kim et al. (2016) found that in first time mothers, lower income was associated with reduced responses to their infant's cry in the medial prefrontal gyrus which is a brain area involved in evaluating the emotional value of stimuli. Additionally, a reduction in responses to the infant cry was found in the middle prefrontal gyrus and superior temporal gyrus which was further associated with less positive perceptions of parenting. These reduced activations were mediated by perceived stress measured in a questionnaire format. This provides more evidence that low income potentially impacts the neurobiological adjustment and neural adaptations to motherhood that enhance a mother's ability to evaluate emotional and social information from infant cues (Kim et al., 2016). This is potentially problematic as a new mother considering infants communicate with their caregivers through their cry. If mothers are less sensitive to this cry due to their brain not properly adapting, they are more likely to not respond to their infant crying. This has large implications for infant health, development, and mother–infant bonding.

4.3 Implications

4.3.1 Implications for Understanding Family Resilience

The capacity of children to maintain functioning in the face of major life stress, being resilient in nature, is largely dependent on their parents as is their risk for living in poverty. Transmission of poverty from parents to their children and future generations often occurs. Individuals who grow up in poor families are more likely to be poor in early adulthood and the chances of being poor in early adulthood increases dramatically as the time spent living in poverty during childhood increases (Wagmiller & Adelman, 2009). Tackling chronic poverty, undertaking childhood poverty and the mechanisms through which the transmission of poverty occurs between generations is of utmost importance.

We reviewed earlier how poverty and related chronic stress influence the health and well-being of both parents and children. These may be some of the key mechanisms underlying the intergenerational transmission of poverty. We suggest the impact of poverty on two generations should be considered for promoting resilience in families. Supporting parents in managing their stress and hardships will allow them to thrive as individuals, manifesting in better every day parenting practices. Coping strategies, attitudes, and aspirations are all items that parents may transmit to their children which could break or maintain poverty cycles (Harper, Marcus, & Moore, 2003). Parents determined to make the most of educational opportunities, work with their children on schoolwork, and educational activities resulted in improved math and reading achievement in low-income African-American families (Datcher-Loury, 1989). Positive parenting and parental investment are two critical strategies that could end the viscous cycle of poverty.

A study following children who were at risk found that two-thirds developed into caring and efficacious adults by the age of 32 (Werner & Smith, 1992), demonstrating that certain factors protect at-risk children from dysfunction. Research has shown that the following factors are present in resilient children: early bonding with a caregiver, mothers who had steady employment, strict parental supervision, good positive coping skills, and enjoyment of school among a long list of other qualities (Benard & Marshall, 1997; Bogenschneider, 1996; Butler, 1997; Hawley & DeHaan, 1996; Parker, Cowen, Work, & Wyman, 1990; Rutter, 1979). Thus, parents may play a large role in whether their children are resilient in the face of adversity by ensuring early bonding as caregivers, providing parental supervision, and encouraging their children to exhibit positive coping skills and excel in school. Children with positive coping strategies (e.g., positive thinking, problem solving, emotion regulation) have also been shown to be resilient, thus making sure at a young age these practices are instilled is of crucial importance. In addition, competence, high self-esteem, good impulse control, achievement in and out of school, and better interpersonal skills are all attributes that help children overcome adversity. Thus far, interventions to reduce stress and improve coping in low-income families have been successful in significantly decreasing stress using positive coping strategies in couples (Wadsworth et al., 2011), which in turn helps couples parent with more competency increasing their children's well-being.

4.3.2 Implications for Practice and Policy

Interventions and policies that adapt a two-generation approach focused on addressing both the needs of parents and children are desirable. In existing programs, for parents, the focus has been supporting effective ways to interact with their children, implementing adaptive coping strategies, and increasing employability. For children, the focus has been enhancing their cognitive control competence as well as learning adaptive coping strategies. Parenting programs similar to Legacy for Children™, Triple P, and Nurse Family Partnership are examples of existing programs that assist parents with engaging in nurturing practices among their children revealing positive impacts; increasing not only parental well-being but also parent–child interactions in families living in poverty (Morris et al., 2017).

Interventions teaching children and parents living in poverty proper coping strategies to manage stress have had positive impacts on families. Reductions in psychological disorders and symptoms as a result of enrollment in coping-based programs such as Coping Cat (Kendall, 1992) and Primary Secondary Control Enhancement Training (Weisz, Thurber, Sweeney, Proffitt, & LeGagnoux, 1997) provide evidence that advanced coping skills are teachable and effective. A pilot study expanded on this work and specifically studied children 8–12 years old and their parents (96% of parents were the mothers of the children). The parent–child dyads participated in a 4 week, 12 hour long pilot prevention program aimed at enhancing coping skills. Children's ability to generate positive coping thoughts and solutions to problems improved from pre- to post-intervention. Additionally, both parents and children had decreases in their involuntary engagement stress response and parents secondary control coping (e.g., cognitive restructuring, positive thinking) increased. Children's internalizing and externalizing symptoms decreased pre- to post-intervention based on parent report (Raviv & Wadsworth, 2010).

Families at risk due to poverty enrolled in interventions that aim to increase positive parent–child interactions and assist with social support through group interventions have shown positive outcomes. Family Check-Up, a home visiting program that assists parents in becoming more positive in their parenting practices found decreases in depressive symptoms (Shaw, Connell, Dishion, Wilson, & Gardner, 2009), decreases in externalizing and internalizing problems in their children (Shaw et al., 2009) compared to controls, and the program is effective in not only families living in poverty but those with other risk factors (Dishion et al., 2008). Another example of a successful intervention is Triple P-Positive Parenting Program, a multi-dimensional program designed to support parenting competence and prevent poor parenting practices. Compared to controls, parents enrolled in the program experienced better well-being, parenting skills (Nowak & Heinrichs, 2008), less stress, depression, and use of forcible parenting (Sanders et al., 2008). Reductions in problem behavior in their children (Nowak & Heinrichs, 2008) and reduced behavioral and emotional problems were also documented (Sanders et al., 2008).

Last, intervention programs of the two-generation approach demonstrated greater positive impacts on child outcomes compared to a child-focused intervention program (Neville et al., 2013). In one family-based program, parents participated in workshops focused on parenting skills and stress regulation while children participated in attention and emotion control training. When compared to a program targeting only children, children of the family-based program showed enhanced neural functions during an attentional control task as well as improved behavioral regulation. This further supports the effectiveness and significance of supporting both generations in the family unit to reduce the intergenerational transmission of poverty.

Breakout Box 4.1: Implications for Practice

I am the managing director for the Birth through Eight Strategy for Tulsa (BEST). I am spearheading efforts to implement a strategy focused on tackling intergenerational poverty by creating a seamless, integrated, and comprehensive continuum of care for the first eight years of a child's life. One of the things that makes it both an exciting job and a job that seems feasible is it's GKFF (George Kaiser Family Foundation) working in collaboration with dozens of public and nonprofit partners across Tulsa to make this possible. It's the only way it can work, because we are talking about a lot of different health, education, and social service providers coming together to offer what they're doing currently to make the services higher quality and integrated for the benefit of the families. Poverty is a complex issue that can affect children and families in a lot of different ways. We know from brain science that those first years of life are a time when a lot of the brain is being developed and, in a positive way, we have an opportunity, during those eight years, and in particular in the first three years, to support positive brain development in a way that is going to help the child realize his or her potential. The circumstances of poverty, like perhaps not having enough food to eat or having challenges in the home related to economic security and physical health, can create challenges for the child's development because in order to really grow and develop in healthy ways...in ways that really reflect the child's potential...there needs to be a certain amount of consistency and security for that child, as well as stimulation. Poverty can create barriers to that kind of environment being around the child for those critical years of development.

I think that in any kind of environment you could have strong or weak relationships between a parent and their child. There are certain things about poverty that might make it more challenging for a parent to develop that strong relationship if they have a lot of concerns and stressors of their own; but that doesn't mean it is a forgone conclusion that the those circumstances will lead to weak relationships or the child not developing in healthy ways. What we're trying to do through BEST is create a lot of different channels for parents to learn about how they can support their child's development, how important these early years are, and from those efforts lay a more solid foundation for the kids. So, it starts in the delivery room where every mom who gives birth is visited by a nurse that carries with her a message about how the mom can support her child's development. We also have home visitation programs targeted at low-income families and different supports through WIC clinics, pediatric well visits, and all these different places where parents are going to be with their young kids in those earliest and most critical stages of development.

The whole emphasis on early childhood and in particular birth through three, comes out of what we learned from brain science, and just how much of the brain is developed in those early years and all the opportunities we have through different initiatives to influence the connections that are made in that child's brain early on. We also look at research and evidence to figure out what programs are going to be supported. Some of them are evidence based programs that may have been from here or in other places, like Durham Connects. From Durham Connects in North Carolina, we brought Family Connects, a home visitation program here. In other cases it could be different initiatives that draw from promising practices in the research, because you don't always have a solid base of evidence to say you know this is going to have an impact on a particular program. On the other hand, there could be elements of other research that convince you that this is a program worth supporting. We also engage in research on an ongoing basis to see how things are working for the children and families that are here in Tulsa. So right now we are looking at how the implementation and ramp up is going. Over time we are going to be looking more closely at the outcomes and impact of our different initiatives on children's development.

—*Sophia Pappas, Managing Director of Birth through Eight Strategy Tulsa*

4.4 Conclusion and Future Directions

Living in poverty may have large impacts on the well-being and health of parents and their children. Parents who experienced harsh parenting and overall received poor quality of parental care during their childhood or experienced chronic stress such as poverty are more likely to show reduced sensitivity to their children and repeat the same parenting practices of their parents. This intergenerational transmission of poverty's negative impacts on parenting therefore needs to be addressed at not only the child's level but the parent's as well. Fostering family resilience in the face of adversity through education about the dangers certain parenting choices may have on the development of children is pivotal.

Research examining how effective the two-generational approach to intervention is, taking into account the well-being of parents and their children, specifically in its ability to build resilience to adversity in the family and stop intergenerational transmission of poverty to future offspring is needed. Intervention at the parent and child level has rarely been studied to our knowledge. Examining the role of resilience on the neural regulation of emotion in both new parents and children living in poverty may provide evidence to support programs intervening using a two-generation approach.

Questions for Thought and Discussion

1. The authors propose that interventions targeting two generations, both parents and their children may help families become more resilient to poverty. Little research currently exists on parents (both mothers and fathers) and their children being involved in such interventions. How would you design a study that would include both generations? What practices would the intervention group undergo to make families more resilient and help eliminate the negative impacts poverty may have?
2. As outlined in this chapter, research supports that poverty may have very negative impacts on the health and mental well-being of parents and their children. Why it is that even in well-developed, wealthy nations such as the United States, poverty is an overwhelming issue? What do you believe needs to happen to help implement policies to eradicate poverty? What are some things you can do at the community level to help?
3. Think of an example of when you faced an adverse situation. How did you effectively cope with the situation? Explain your thought process of coping with the situation with a partner. How would you translate your coping skill set to an at-risk group? What are some simple ways to describe your coping strategies? What would you use to illustrate your points and effectively teach your coping methods?
4. In March of 2015 the following headline appeared in the Scientific American, *Poverty Shrinks Brain from Birth*. This headline was based off of research done by Dr. Kimberly Noble and colleagues published in Nature Neuroscience, an article discussed in this chapter. What are some potential issues you see with this headline? Do you see any risks in publishing findings suggesting this? In what ways could neurobiological research of this nature effectively inform policy? How might someone living in poverty perceive this headline?

Glossary

Allostatic load The physiological consequence of chronic exposure to fluctuating or heightened neural or neuroendocrine responses that result from repeated or chronic stress resulting in "wear and tear" on the body.

Amygdala An almond-shaped mass of gray matter in each cerebral hemisphere of the brain involved in experiencing emotions.

Coping The process of adapting to stress that includes conscious attempts to manage emotions to face and deal with problems, stress, difficulties, or challenges in an effective and successful manner.

Cortisol A steroid hormone produced by the adrenal cortex involved in metabolism and helps us regulate stress within the body.

Cumulative stress The accumulation of mental and/or emotional strain/tension resulting from multiple adverse or very demanding circumstances (e.g., heavy workload, multiple frustrations).

Depression A mood disorder, also called major depressive disorder or clinical depression, which causes a persistent feeling of sadness and loss of interest. It affects how you feel, think, and behave and can lead to a variety of emotional and physical problems.

Hippocampus Curved elongated ridges on the floor of each lateral ventricle in the brain thought to be involved in the formation, storage, and processing of memories.

Income-to-needs ratio The ratio of family or unrelated individuals' combined income relative to the appropriate poverty threshold. Ratios below 1.00 indicate that the income for the family or unrelated individuals is below the poverty line, whereas a ratio above 1.00 indicates income above the poverty line.

Intergenerational poverty Poverty induced by the socially and/or economically challenged background of a person's parents.

Intergenerational transmission of parenting Process by which unintendedly or purposively an earlier generation psychologically influences parenting attitudes and behavior of the next generation.

Neural sensitivity The fraction of neurons that show positive responses to a stimulus.

Positive parenting Warm, responsive, sensitive, and consistent parenting that provides boundaries and contingent limits for children in a low-conflict family environment.

Poverty The state or condition of lacking a socially acceptable amount of money or material possessions.

Socioeconomic disadvantage Individuals who have limited access to materials and/or resources which impacts their ability to participate in society.

Socioeconomic status Social standing of an individual or group, often measured as a combination of education, income, and occupation.

Telomeres Repetitive sequences of DNA that do not code for proteins, but function as caps at the end of each strand of DNA that protect our chromosomes.

References

Azad, M. B., Lissitsyn, Y., Miller, G. E., Becker, A. B., HayGlass, K. T., & Kozyrskyj, A. L. (2012). Influence of socioeconomic status trajectories on innate immune responsiveness in children. *PLoS One, 7*, e38669. https://doi.org/10.1371/journal.pone.0038669

Barch, D., Pagliaccio, D., Belden, A., Harms, M. P., Gaffrey, M., Sylvester, C. M., … Luby, J. (2016). Effect of hippocampal and amygdala connectivity on the relationship between preschool poverty and school-age depression. *American Journal of Psychiatry, 173*, 625–634. https://doi.org/10.1176/appi.ajp.2015.15081014

Barrett, J., & Fleming, A. S. (2011). Annual research review: All mothers are not created equal: Neural and psychobiological perspectives on mothering and the importance of individual differences. *Journal of Child Psychology and Psychiatry, 52*, 368–397. https://doi.org/10.1111/j.1469-7610.2010.02306.x

Belsky, J., Pasco Fearon, R., & Bell, B. (2007). Parenting, attention and externalizing problems: Testing mediation longitudinally, repeatedly and reciprocally. *Journal of Child Psychology and Psychiatry, 48*, 1233–1242. https://doi.org/10.1111/j.1469-7610.2007.01807.x

Benard, B., & Marshall, K. (1997). A framework for practice: Tapping innate resilience. *Research/Practice, 5*, 9–15.

Benasich, A. A., Gou, Z., Choudhury, N., & Harris, K. D. (2008). Early cognitive and language skills are linked to resting frontal gamma power across the first 3 years. *Behavioural Brain Research, 195*, 215–222. https://doi.org/10.1016/j.bbr.2008.08.049

Blair, C., Berry, D., Mills-Koonce, R., & Granger, D. (2013). Cumulative effects of early poverty on cortisol in young children: Moderation by autonomic nervous system activity. *Psychoneuroendocrinology, 38*, 2666–2675. https://doi.org/10.1016/j.psyneuen.2013.06.025

Bogenschneider, K. (1996). An ecological risk/protective theory for building prevention programs, policies, and community capacity to support youth. *Family Relations, 45*, 127–138. https://doi.org/10.2307/585283

Bradley, R. H., & Corwyn, R. F. (2002). Socioeconomic status and child development. *Annual Review of Psychology, 53*, 371–399. https://doi.org/10.1146/annurev.psych.53.100901.135233

Brody, G. H., Lei, M.-K., Chen, E., & Miller, G. E. (2014). Neighborhood poverty and allostatic load in African American youth. *Pediatrics, 134*, e1362–e1368. https://doi.org/10.1542/peds.2014-1395

Bus, A. G., Van Ijzendoorn, M. H., & Pellegrini, A. D. (1995). Joint book reading makes for success in learning to read: A meta-analysis on intergenerational transmission of literacy. *Review of Educational Research, 6*, 1–21. https://doi.org/10.3102/00346543065001001

Butler, K. (1997). The anatomy of resilience. *Family Therapy Networker, 21*, 22–27.

Chapman, D. P., Dube, S. R., & Anda, R. F. (2007). Adverse childhood events as risk factors for negative mental health outcomes. *Psychiatric Annals, 37*, 355–364.

Chen, E., Hanson, M. D., Paterson, L. Q., Griffin, M. J., Walker, H. A., & Miller, G. E. (2006). Socioeconomic status and inflammatory processes in childhood asthma: The role of psychological stress. *Journal of Allergy and Clinical Immunology, 11*, 1014–1020. https://doi.org/10.1016/j.jaci.2006.01.036

Chen, E., Matthews, K. A., & Boyce, W. T. (2002). Socioeconomic differences in children's health: How and why do these relationships change with age? *Psychological Bulletin, 12*, 295–329. https://doi.org/10.1037//0033-2909.128.2.295

Conger, R. D., Ge, X., Elder, G. H., Lorenz, F. O., & Simons, R. L. (1994). Economic stress, coercive family process, and developmental problems of adolescents. *Child Development, 65*, 541–561. https://doi.org/10.2307/1131401

Datcher-Loury, L. (1989). Family background and school achievement among low income blacks. *Journal of Human Resources, 24*, 528–544. https://doi.org/10.2307/145826

Dishion, T. J., Shaw, D., Connell, A., Gardner, F., Weaver, C., & Wilson, M. (2008). The family check-up with high-risk indigent families: Preventing problem behavior by increasing parents' positive behavior support in early childhood. *Child Development, 79*, 1395–1414. https://doi.org/10.1111/j.1467-8624.2008.01195.x

Dohrenwend, B. S. (1973). Social status and stressful life events. *Journal of Personality and Social Psychology, 28*, 225–235. https://doi.org/10.1037/h0035718

Drury, S. S., Mabile, E., Brett, Z. H., Esteves, K., Jones, E., Shirtcliff, E. A., & Theall, K. P. (2014). The association of telomere length with family violence and disruption. *Pediatrics, 134*, e128–e137. https://doi.org/10.1542/peds.2013-3415

Duncan, G. J., Brooks-Gunn, J., & Klebanov, P. K. (1994). Economic deprivation and early childhood development. *Child Development, 65*, 296–318. https://doi.org/10.2307/1131385

Earls, F., McGuire, J., & Shay, S. (1994). Evaluating a community intervention to reduce the risk of child abuse: Methodological strategies in conducting neighborhood surveys. *Child Abuse & Neglect, 18*, 473–485. https://doi.org/10.1016/0145-2134(94)90031-0

Eisenberg, N. (2008). Understanding mother-adolescent conflict discussions: Concurrent and across-time prediction from youths' dispositions and parenting. *Monographs of the Society for Reseach in Child Development, 73*, vii–viii, 1–160. https://doi.org/10.1111/j.1540-5834.2008.00470.x

Essex, M. J., Klein, M. H., Cho, E., & Kalin, N. H. (2002). Maternal stress beginning in infancy may sensitize children to later stress exposure: Effects on cortisol and behavior. *Biological Psychiatry, 52*, 776–784. https://doi.org/10.1016/s0006-3223(02)01553-6

Evans, G. W. (2004). The environment of childhood poverty. *American Psychologist, 59*, 77–92. https://doi.org/10.1037/0003-066X.59.2.77

Evans, G. W., Chen, E., Miller, G., & Seeman, T. (2012). How poverty gets under the skin: A life course perspective. In V. Maholmes & R. King (Eds.), *The Oxford handbook of poverty and child development* (pp. 13–36). Oxford, UK: Oxford University Press. https://doi.org/10.1093/oxfordhb/9780199769100.013.0001

Evans, G. W., & English, K. (2002). The environment of poverty: Multiple stressor exposure, psychophysiological stress, and socioemotional adjustment. *Child Development, 73*, 1238–1248. https://doi.org/10.1111/1467-8624.00469

Evans, G. W., & Kim, P. (2007). Childhood poverty and health: Cumulative risk exposure and stress dysregulation. *Psychological Science, 18*, 953–957. https://doi.org/10.1111/j.1467-9280.2007.02008.x

Farah, M. J., Shera, D. M., Savage, J. H., Betancourt, L., Giannetta, J. M., Brodsky, N. L., … Hurt, H. (2006). Childhood poverty: Specific associations with neurocognitive development. *Brain Research, 1110*, 166–174. https://doi.org/10.1016/j.brainres.2006.06.072

Field, T. (2010). Postpartum depression effects on early interactions, parenting, and safety practices: A review. *Infant Behavior and Development, 33*, 1–6. https://doi.org/10.1016/j.infbeh.2009.10.005

Flinn, M. V., & England, B. G. (1997). Social economics of childhood glucocorticoid stress response and health. *American Journal of Physical Anthropology, 102*, 33–53. https://doi.org/10.1002/(sici)1096-8644(199701)102:13.3.co;2-u.

Furstenberg, F. F., Belzer, A., Davis, C., Levine, J. A., Morrow, K., & Washington, M. (1993). How families manage risk and opportunity in dangerous neighborhoods. *Sociology and the Public Agenda, 8*, 231–258. https://doi.org/10.4135/9781483325484.n12

Ganzel, B. L., Kim, P., Gilmore, H., Tottenham, N., & Temple, E. (2013). Stress and the healthy adolescent brain: Evidence for the neural embedding of life events. *Development and Psychopathology, 25*, 879–889. https://doi.org/10.1017/s0954579413000242

Gao, W., Alcauter, S., Elton, A., Hernandez-Castillo, C. R., Smith, J. K., Ramirez, J., & Lin, W. (2015). Functional network development during the first year: Relative sequence and socioeconomic correlations. *Cerebral Cortex, 25*, 2919–2928. https://doi.org/10.1093/cercor/bhu088

Gelles, R. J. (1992). Poverty and violence toward children. *American Behavioral Scientist, 35*, 258–274. https://doi.org/10.1177/0002764292035003005

Gianaros, P. J., Horenstein, J. A., Hariri, A. R., Sheu, L. K., Manuck, S. B., Matthews, K. A., & Cohen, S. (2008). Potential neural embedding of parental social standing. *Social Cognitive and Affective Neuroscience, 3*, 91–96. https://doi.org/10.1093/scan/nsn003

Gilman, S. E., Kawachi, I., Fitzmaurice, G. M., & Buka, S. L. (2002). Socioeconomic status in childhood and the lifetime risk of major depression. *International Journal of Epidemiology, 31*, 359–367. https://doi.org/10.1093/ije/31.2.359

Goodman, E., McEwen, B. S., Huang, B., Dolan, L. M., & Adler, N. E. (2005). Social inequalities in biomarkers of cardiovascular risk in adolescence. *Psychosomatic Medicine, 67*, 9–15. https://doi.org/10.1097/01.psy.0000149254.36133.1a

Goyal, D., Gay, C., & Lee, K. A. (2010). How much does low socioeconomic status increase the risk of prenatal and postpartum depressive symptoms in first-time mothers? *Women's Health Issues, 20*, 96–104. https://doi.org/10.1016/j.whi.2009.11.003

Gustafsson, P. E., Gustafsson, P. A., & Nelson, N. (2006). Cortisol levels and psychosocial factors in preadolescent children. *Stress and Health, 22*, 3–9. https://doi.org/10.1002/smi.1074

Hair, N. L., Hanson, J. L., Wolfe, B. L., & Pollak, S. D. (2015). Association of child poverty, brain development, and academic achievement. *JAMA Pediatrics, 169*, 822–829. https://doi.org/10.1001/jamapediatrics.2015.1475

Harper, C., Marcus, R., & Moore, K. (2003). Enduring poverty and the conditions of childhood: Lifecourse and intergenerational poverty transmissions. *World Development, 31*, 535–554. https://doi.org/10.1016/s0305-750x(03)00010-x

Hawley, D. R., & DeHaan, L. (1996). Toward a definition of family resilience: Integrating life-span and family perspectives. *Family Process, 35*, 283–298. https://doi.org/10.1111/j.1545-5300.1996.00283.x

Howard, E. C. (2000). *Employment, social support, and well-being among low-income mothers: A qualitative and quantitative analysis*. Evanston, IL: Northwestern University.

Jarrett, R. L. (1997). Bringing families back in: Neighborhood effects on child development. *Neighborhood Poverty, 2*, 48–64.

Kendall, P. C. (1992). *Coping cat workbook*. Ardmore, PA: Woorkbook Publishing.

Kim, P., & Bianco, H. (2014). Understanding how motherhood and poverty change the brain. *Zero to Three, 34*, 29–36.

Kim, P., Capistrano, C., & Congleton, C. (2016). Socioeconomic disadvantages and neural sensitivity to infant cry: Role of maternal distress. *Social Cognitive and Affective Neuroscience, 11*, 1597–1607. https://doi.org/10.1093/scan/nsw063

Kim, P., Leckman, J. F., Mayes, L. C., Feldman, R., Wang, X., & Swain, J. E. (2010). The plasticity of human maternal brain: Longitudinal changes in brain anatomy during the early postpartum period. *Behavioral Neuroscience, 124*, 695–700. https://doi.org/10.1037/a0020884

Kishiyama, M. M., Boyce, W. T., Jimenez, A. M., Perry, L. M., & Knight, R. T. (2009). Socioeconomic disparities affect prefrontal function in children. *Journal of Cognitive Neuroscience, 21*, 1106–1115. https://doi.org/10.1162/jocn.2009.21101

Kollerud, R. D. R., Blaasaas, K. G., & Claussen, B. (2015). Poverty and the risk of leukemia and cancer in the central nervous system in children: A cohort study in a high-income country. *Scandinavian Journal of Public Health, 43*, 736–743. https://doi.org/10.1177/1403494815590499

Lugo-Gil, J., & Tamis-LeMonda, C. S. (2008). Family resources and parenting quality: Links to children's cognitive development across the first 3 years. *Child Development, 79*, 1065–1085. https://doi.org/10.1111/j.1467-8624.2008.01176.x

Lupien, S. J., King, S., Meaney, M. J., & McEwen, B. S. (2000). Child's stress hormone levels correlate with mother's socioeconomic status and depressive state. *Biological Psychiatry, 48*, 976–980. https://doi.org/10.1016/s0006-3223(00)00965-3

Lupien, S. J., King, S., Meaney, M. J., & McEwen, B. S. (2001). Can poverty get under your skin? Basal cortisol levels and cognitive function in children from low and high socioeconomic status. *Development and Psychopathology, 13*, 653–676. https://doi.org/10.1017/s0954579401003133

Mackey, A. P., Finn, A. S., Leonard, J. A., Jacoby-Senghor, D. S., West, M. R., Gabrieli, C. F., & Gabrieli, J. D. (2015). Neuroanatomical correlates of the income-achievement gap. *Psychological Science, 26*, 925–933. https://doi.org/10.1177/0956797615572233

Magnuson, K. A., & Duncan, G. J. (2002). Parents in poverty. *Handbook of Parenting, 4*, 95–121.

Malcolm, C., MacKay, W., Shepherd, A., & Weaver, L. (2004). Helicobacter pylori in children is strongly associated with poverty. *Scottish Medical Journal, 49*, 136–138. https://doi.org/10.1177/003693300404900406

Massey, D. S., & Eggers, M. L. (1990). The ecology of inequality: Minorities and the concentration of poverty, 1970–1980. *American Journal of Sociology, 95*, 1153–1188. https://doi.org/10.1086/229425

McCloskey, L. A., Figueredo, A. J., & Koss, M. P. (1995). The effects of systemic family violence on children's mental health. *Child Development, 66*, 1239–1261. https://doi.org/10.2307/1131645

McLeod, J. D., & Shanahan, M. J. (1993). Poverty, parenting, and children's mental health. *American Sociological Review*, 351–366. https://doi.org/10.2307/2095905

Miller, G. E., & Chen, E. (2013). The biological residue of childhood poverty. *Child Development Perspectives, 7*, 67–73. https://doi.org/10.1111/cdep.12021

Miller, J. E., & Korenman, S. (1994). Poverty and children's nutritional status in the United States. *American Journal of Epidemiology, 140*, 233–243. https://doi.org/10.1093/oxfordjournals.aje.a117242

Mitchell, C., Hobcraft, J., McLanahan, S. S., Siegel, S. R., Berg, A., Brooks-Gunn, J., … Notterman, D. (2014). Social disadvantage, genetic sensitivity, and children's telomere length. *Proceedings of the National Academy of Sciences, 111*, 5944–5949. https://doi.org/10.1073/pnas.1404293111

Morris, A. S., Robinson, L. R., Hays-Grudo, J., Claussen, A. H., Hartwig, S. A., & Treat, A. E. (2017). Targeting parenting in early childhood: A public health approach to improve outcomes for children living in poverty. *Child Development, 88*, 388–397. https://doi.org/10.1111/cdev.12743

Murray, L. (1992). The impact of postnatal depression on infant development. *Journal of Child Psychology and Psychiatry, 33*, 543–561. https://doi.org/10.1111/j.1469-7610.1992.tb00890.x

Muscatell, K. A., Morelli, S. A., Falk, E. B., Way, B. M., Pfeifer, J. H., Galinsky, A. D., … Eisenberger, N. I. (2012). Social status modulates neural activity in the mentalizing network. *Neuroimage, 60*, 1771–1777. https://doi.org/10.1016/j.neuroimage.2012.01.080

Neville, H. J., Stevens, C., Pakulak, E., Bell, T. A., Fanning, J., Klein, S., & Isbell, E. (2013). Family-based training program improves brain function, cognition, and behavior in lower socioeconomic status preschoolers. *Proceedings of the National Academy of Sciences, 110*, 12138–12143. https://doi.org/10.1073/pnas.1304437110

Newland, R. P., Crnic, K. A., Cox, M. J., & Mills-Koonce, W. R. (2013). The family model stress and maternal psychological symptoms: Mediated pathways from economic hardship to parenting. *Journal of Family Psychology, 27*, 96–105. https://doi.org/10.1037/a0031112

Noble, K. G., Houston, S. M., Brito, N. H., Bartsch, H., Kan, E., Kuperman, J. M., … Libiger, O. (2015). Family income, parental education and brain structure in children and adolescents. *Nature Neuroscience, 18*, 773–778. https://doi.org/10.1038/nn.3983

Noble, K. G., Houston, S. M., Kan, E., & Sowell, E. R. (2012). Neural correlates of socioeconomic status in the developing human brain. *Developmental Science, 15*, 516–527. https://doi.org/10.1111/j.1467-7687.2012.01147.x

Nowak, C., & Heinrichs, N. (2008). A comprehensive meta-analysis of triple P-positive parenting program using hierarchical linear modeling: Effectiveness and moderating variables. *Clinical Child and Family Psychology Review, 11*, 114–144. https://doi.org/10.1007/s10567-008-0033-0

Ogden, C. L., Lamb, M. M., Carroll, M. D., & Flegal, K. M. (2010). Obesity and socioeconomic status in children and adolescents: United States, 2005–2008. NCHS Data Brief. Number 51. *National Center for Health Statistics*.

Paneth, N. S. (1995). The problem of low birth weight. *The Future of Children, 5*, 19–34. https://doi.org/10.2307/1602505

Parker, G. R., Cowen, E. L., Work, W. C., & Wyman, P. A. (1990). Test correlates of stress resilience among urban school children. *Journal of Primary Prevention, 11*, 19–35. https://doi.org/10.1007/bf01324859

Pinderhughes, E. E., Nix, R., Foster, E. M., & Jones, D. (2001). Parenting in context: Impact of neighborhood poverty, residential stability, public services, social networks, and danger on parental behaviors. *Journal of Marriage and Family, 63*, 941–953. https://doi.org/10.1111/j.1741-3737.2001.00941.x

Rainisch, B. K. W., & Upchurch, D. M. (2013). Sociodemographic correlates of allostatic load among a national sample of adolescents: Findings from the National Health and Nutrition Examination Survey, 1999–2008. *Journal of Adolescent Health, 53*, 506–511. https://doi.org/10.1016/j.jadohealth.2013.04.020

Raviv, T., & Wadsworth, M. E. (2010). The efficacy of a pilot prevention program for children and caregivers coping with economic strain. *Cognitive Therapy and Research, 34*, 216–228. https://doi.org/10.1007/s10608-009-9265-7

Rutter, M. (1979). Protective factors in children's responses to stress and disadvantage. *Annals of the Academy of Medicine, Singapore, 8*, 324–338.

Sanders, M. R., Ralph, A., Sofronoff, K., Gardiner, P., Thompson, R., Dwyer, S., & Bidwell, K. (2008). Every family: A population approach to reducing behavioral and emotional problems in children making the transition to school. *The Journal of Primary Prevention, 29*, 197–222. https://doi.org/10.1007/s10935-008-0139-7

Seeman, T., Epel, E., Gruenewald, T., Karlamangla, A., & McEwen, B. S. (2010). Socio-economic differentials in peripheral biology: Cumulative allostatic load. *Annals of the New York Academy of Sciences, 1186*, 223–239. https://doi.org/10.1111/j.1749-6632.2009.05341.x

Shammas, M. A. (2011). Telomeres, lifestyle, cancer, and aging. *Current Opinion in Clinical Nutrition and Metabolic Care, 14*, 28. https://doi.org/10.1097/MCO.0b013e32834121b1

Shaw, D. S., Connell, A., Dishion, T. J., Wilson, M. N., & Gardner, F. (2009). Improvements in maternal depression as a mediator of intervention effects on early childhood problem behavior. *Development and Psychopathology, 21*, 417–439. https://doi.org/10.1017/s0954579409000236

Sheridan, M. A., Sarsour, K., Jutte, D., D'Esposito, M., & Boyce, W. T. (2012). The impact of social disparity on prefrontal function in childhood. *PLoS One, 7*, e35744. https://doi.org/10.1371/journal.pone.0035744

Simons, R. L., Johnson, C., Conger, R. D., & Lorenz, F. O. (1997). Linking community context to quality of parenting: A study of rural families. *Rural Sociology, 62*, 207–230. https://doi.org/10.1111/j.1549-0831.1997.tb00651.x

Smith, J. R., Brooks-Gunn, J., & Klebanov, P. K. (1997). Consequences of living in poverty for young children's cognitive and verbal ability and early school achievement. *Consequences of Growing Up Poor*, 132–189.

Sobal, J., & Stunkard, A. J. (1989). Socioeconomic status and obesity: A review of the literature. *Psychological Bulletin, 105*, 260–275. https://doi.org/10.1037//0033-2909.105.2.260

Stepnowsky, C. J., Jr., Nelesen, R. A., DeJardin, D., & Dimsdale, J. E. (2004). Socioeconomic status is associated with nocturnal blood pressure dipping. *Psychosomatic Medicine, 66*, 651–655. https://doi.org/10.1097/01.psy.0000138124.58216.6c

Swain, J. E., Kim, P., Spicer, J., Ho, S., Dayton, C. J., Elmadih, A., & Abel, K. (2014). Approaching the biology of human parental attachment: Brain imaging, oxytocin and coordinated assessments of mothers and fathers. *Brain Research, 1580*, 78–101. https://doi.org/10.1016/j.brainres.2014.03.007

Tomalski, P., Moore, D. G., Ribeiro, H., Axelsson, E. L., Murphy, E., Karmiloff-Smith, A., … Kushnerenko, E. (2013). Socioeconomic status and functional brain development—Associations in early infancy. *Developmental Science, 16*, 676–687. https://doi.org/10.1111/desc.12079

van Oort, F. V., van der Ende, J., Wadsworth, M. E., Verhulst, F. C., & Achenbach, T. M. (2011). Cross-national comparison of the link between socioeconomic status and emotional and behavioral problems in youths. *Social Psychiatry and Psychiatric Epidemiology, 46*, 167–172. https://doi.org/10.1007/s00127-010-0191-5

Vliegenthart, J., Noppe, G., van Rossum, E., Koper, J., Raat, H., & van den Akker, E. (2016). Socioeconomic status in children is associated with hair cortisol levels as a biological measure of chronic stress. *Psychoneuroendocrinology, 65*, 9–14. https://doi.org/10.1016/j.psyneuen.2015.11.022

Wadsworth, M. E., Santiago, C. D., Einhorn, L., Etter, E. M., Rienks, S., & Markman, H. (2011). Preliminary efficacy of an intervention to reduce psychosocial stress and improve coping in low-income families. *American Journal of Community Psychology, 48*, 257–271. https://doi.org/10.1007/s10464-010-9384-z

Wagmiller, R. L., & Adelman, R. M. (2009). Childhood and intergenerational poverty: The long-term consequences of growing up poor. *Columbia University Academic Commons*. https://doi.org/10.7916/D8MP5C0Z

Walker, L., Timmerman, G. M., Kim, M., & Sterling, B. (2002). Relationships between body image and depressive symptoms during postpartum in ethnically diverse, low income women. *Women & Health, 36*, 101–121. https://doi.org/10.1300/J013v36n03_07

Wang, Y., & Zhang, Q. (2006). Are American children and adolescents of low socioeconomic status at increased risk of obesity? Changes in the association between overweight and family income between 1971 and 2002. *The American Journal of Clinical Nutrition, 84*, 707–716. https://doi.org/10.1093/ajcn/84.4.707

Weisz, J. R., Thurber, C. A., Sweeney, L., Proffitt, V. D., & LeGagnoux, G. L. (1997). Brief treatment of mild-to-moderate child depression using primary and secondary control enhancement training. *Journal of Consulting and Clinical Psychology, 65*, 703–707. https://doi.org/10.1037/0022-006X.65.4.703

Werner, E. E., & Smith, R. S. (1992). *Overcoming the odds: High risk children from birth to adulthood*. Cornell, NY: Cornell University Press.

Wilson, D. K., Kliewer, W., Plybon, L., & Sica, D. A. (2000). Socioeconomic status and blood pressure reactivity in healthy black adolescents. *Hypertension, 35*, 496–500. https://doi.org/10.1161/01.hyp.35.1.496

Wilson, W. J. (1987). *The truly disadvantaged: The inner city, the underclass, and social policy*. Chicago, IL: University of Chicago Press.

Chapter 5
The Influence of Teacher–Child Relationships on Preschool Children's Cortisol Levels

Bridget E. Hatfield

Early childhood marks a critical period when the relationships and interactions children experience shape all domains of development. For instance, young children learn how to regulate emotions through the process of co-regulation (e.g., rocking a crying child to help soothe), laying the foundations for regulatory strategies the child can use in the future (Bernier, Carlson, & Whipple, 2010). Language develops through exposure to words, conversations, and other mechanisms via interactions with others, and the quality of those conversations is critical to support language development (Hirsh-Pasek et al., 2015). In addition to research, developmental theory also posits that interactions are the driving force of development (Bronfenbrenner & Morris, 2006). Relatedly, interactions and relationships with caregivers also help to shape the developing stress response system.

The stress response system is especially malleable prenatally and throughout early childhood (Meaney et al., 1996). In particular, the hypothalamic pituitary adrenal (HPA) axis, one component of the stress response system, is influenced by aspects of the environment including child–caregiver relationships (Loman, Gunnar, and The Early Experience, Stress, and Neurobehavioral Development Center, 2010). Experimental research with animals indicates that early caregiving has generational effects, altering gene expression and behavior (Meaney, 2001). In humans, correlational research investigating the importance of relationships on the HPA axis is abundant, with most highlighting that responsive, sensitive, and long-term positive relationships have lasting effects on HPA axis functioning, particularly in early childhood (Gunnar & Donzella, 2002; Meaney et al., 1996). Beyond the family, interactions with teachers in early care and education (ECE) settings also help shape young children's HPA axis.

B. E. Hatfield (✉)
College of Public Health and Human Sciences, School of Social and Behavioral Health Sciences, Oregon State University, Corvallis, OR, USA
e-mail: bridget.hatfield@oregonstate.edu

A. W. Harrist, B. C. Gardner (eds.), *Biobehavioral Markers in Risk and Resilience Research*, Emerging Issues in Family and Individual Resilience,
https://doi.org/10.1007/978-3-030-05952-1_5

Sixty-one percent of children under the age of five are enrolled in some type of ECE program (Laughlin, 2013), constituting the ECE environment as an important setting that may influence children's health and development. Often, the mechanism through which children's development is supported is the quality of the interactions with teachers, peers, and tasks in the ECE setting. In fact, there is a large body of evidence indicating that high-quality ECE settings contribute to preschool children's school readiness skills, such as language and self-regulatory skills (Burchinal, Vandergift, Pianta, & Mashburn, 2010; Hamre, Hatfield, Pianta, & Jamil, 2014; Weiland, Ulvestad, Sachs, & Yoshikawa, 2013), and in some cases the effect sustains even after accounting for the home environment (e.g., Romano, Kohen, & Findlay, 2010). The importance of ECE settings extends to emerging research focused on understanding how the teacher–child relationship affects children's HPA axis. As with school readiness skills, teacher–child relationships and interactions are associated with young children's functioning in the HPA axis (Hatfield, Hestenes, Kintner-Duffy, & O'Brien, 2013; Lisonbee, Mize, Lapp Payne, & Granger, 2008). This chapter focuses on how the teacher–child relationship affects the developing stress response system in preschool children, with a focus on the HPA axis.

5.1 Child Care Quality and Child Outcomes

Over the past two decades, substantial research across a variety of populations converges on the importance of the ECE environment for children's development. While the home environment and the parent–child relationship is critical and arguably the most important in shaping development (National Academics of Sciences, Engineering, & Medicine, 2016), the relationships and interactions that children experience in ECE are also important contributors to children's development. These programs are also financially beneficial as economic evidence indicates that returns on investment related to attendance in preschool are higher, \$4 to over \$10 return on investment, when the quality of those programs is high (Reynolds & Temple, 2008).

Generally, quality in ECE classrooms is defined in two ways: structural and process quality. Structural quality includes aspects of the classroom like curriculum, teacher education, teacher–child ratio, and materials (Hestenes, Cassidy, Hegde, & Lower, 2007). These foundational aspects, such as teacher–child ratio and teacher education, are related to language and cognition (Burchinal et al., 2000), and there is some evidence that structural quality is related to children's activity in the HPA axis. For example, children who were enrolled in low-structural quality environments experienced elevated cortisol level throughout the day (Sajaniemi et al., 2011). On the other hand, process quality encompasses factors focused on relationships and interactions such as a teacher sensitively responding to a child's question, effectively using the curriculum to facilitate learning, and having language-rich interactions (Mashburn et al., 2008). These types of high-quality teacher–child interactions and relationships are related to host of domains of development (Hamre, 2014), including children's cortisol patterns. The driving force of influence on school readiness skills is process quality although structural quality is thought to lay the foundation for high-process quality (Mashburn et al., 2008).

Given the importance of process quality, a preponderance of research has focused on investigating the associations between child outcomes and process quality, with a focus on high-quality teacher–child interactions and relationships. Overall, children who attend preschool programs that are rated high in sensitive, responsive, and warm teacher–child interactions are more likely to show higher language and literacy skills, are better able to control behaviors and attention, and have more sophisticated social skills than children in classroom with lower quality teacher–child interactions (Burchinal et al., 2008; Hatfield, Burchinal, Pianta, & Sideris, 2016; Soliday Hong, Howes, Marcella, Zucker, & Huang, 2015; Weiland et al., 2013). A recent report agrees that, "Convincing evidence shows that children attending a diverse array of state and school district pre-k programs are more ready for school at the end of their pre-k year than children who do not attend pre-k agreement" (Phillips et al., 2017, p. 9), and quality plays a role in augmenting those pre-k experiences.

At a proximal level, a preschool child with a close teacher–child relationship, compared to those with a conflictual teacher–child relationship, is more likely to show greater school readiness skills. Children who have a close relationship with a teacher are more likely to demonstrate higher levels of self-regulation, language, literacy, and social skills (Birch & Ladd, 1997; Schmidt, Pentimonti, & Justice, 2012). These positive associations between relationships and skills are evident from preschool into high school (Roorda, Koomen, Split, & Oort, 2011). Challenging behaviors are less likely during the preschool year (Howes, 2000) and in subsequent years (Silver, Measelle, Armstrong, & Essex, 2005) when a child has a close teacher–child relationship.

In addition to children, families also benefit from high-quality child care. Families whose children attended Head Start, a highly resourced ECE program, are less likely to engage in spanking (Pratt, Lipscomb, & Schmitt, 2015; Zhai, Waldfogel, & Brooks-Gunn, 2013), and more likely to read and do math activities with their children (Gelber & Isen, 2013). In Germany, mothers of young children who lived in a region with higher quality care were more likely to be employed and work longer hours (Schober & Spiess, 2015). Additionally, families receiving child care subsidies in Massachusetts were more likely to enroll their child in high-quality care (Marshall, Wagner Robeson, Tracy, Frye, & Roberts, 2013), which is promising as use of subsidies promotes long-term employment (Danziger, Ananat, & Browning, 2004) and reduces work-family conflict (Press, Fagan, & Laughlin, 2006).

Beyond correlational research supporting the role of high-quality ECE on children and their families, experimental research indicates causal mechanisms between teacher–child interactions and relationships and children's school readiness skills. A recent meta-analysis revealed that intervention programs designed to promote improved quality of teacher–child interactions in child care have a small to medium effect ($g = .26$) on children's socioemotional development (Wener, Linting, Vermeer, & van IJzeondoorn, 2016). Other programs reveal improvements in preschool children's academic skills; a video-based professional development intervention aimed to increase classroom quality via improved teacher–child interactions shows gains in language (Mashburn, Downer, Hamre, Justice, & Pianta, 2010). Longitudinal studies suggest long-term benefits of high quality ECE programming on adolescent academic achievement (Vandell, Belsky, Burchinal, Steinberg, Vandergrist, and NICHD Early Child Care Research Network, 2010) and higher rates of high school graduation (Ludwig & Miller, 2007).

Breakout Box 5.1: Focus on Practice

As a professional in the field of early childhood for many years, I cannot overstate the importance of teacher–child relationships in the lives of young children and their families. A strong relationship between a caregiver or teacher and a child helps the child learn to connect to others at an early age, which fosters the child's self-regulation and has a positive influence on the child's developmental trajectory. Teachers also benefit from connecting with young children; it gives teachers a sense of purpose and affirmation that they are having an impact on children's lives. Providing early care and education can feel like a thankless job at times; I've seen how intense connections between children and teachers are just as important and rewarding for teachers as they are for children.

I work with children and families who come to us experiencing different types of poverty, including cyclical and temporary poverty. Our families have a broad range of needs, and the goal is to meet families where they are. We always assume the best of our families; we help them find their strengths, then guide them towards accessing and utilizing those strengths to set goals and meet the needs of their children and families. Teachers play a critical role in this process. One particular example of this stands out to me. We had a child who came to our program who was non-verbal. We helped the family access not only ancillary services, but also evaluation and follow-up services; we were also intentional about nurturing the teacher–child relationship. The child's first classroom placement was with a warm, competent teacher, but the child simply didn't connect to the teacher. We moved the child to a different classroom, where the child and teacher formed a strong connection. In fact, the child connected with the teacher in ways that they didn't even connect with the family. The child learned communication skills, which in turn reduced stress and frustration, and enabled the child to interact with peers.

Teachers need tools to be successful in their work with children and families, and this consists of more than simply dumping information into their brains in a professional development workshop. Rather, they need to practice what they are learning, and coaching is essential. Their work is important, and they deserve support. I want teachers to know they are a BIG DEAL. They can make or break a child's love of learning. They can help a child realize they can become anything they want to be. They may not know it at the time, but they will have a tremendous, positive impact on children's lives.

–*Paula Brown*, Mental Health & Disabilities Services Manager for Early Head Start

Given the impact of high-quality preschool programming on children, it is unsurprising that more research extends beyond school readiness skills to health and the stress response system. A recent study found that adolescents who attended preschool (compared to home-based or parent only care) were more likely to have better blood pressure (Sabol & Hoyt, 2017). Positive health benefits seem to persist into adulthood as males who were enrolled in the Abecedarian Preschool project, a high-quality preschool program, had better adult male systolic blood pressure and higher levels of the high-density lipoprotein cholesterol, the "good cholesterol" (Campbell et al., 2014). Regarding activity in the HPA axis, children in ECE may be at risk for elevated cortisol patterns while attending child care (Sabol & Hoyt, 2017; Vermeer & van Ijzendoorn, 2006); however, positive teacher–child relationships may mitigate this aberrant pattern (e.g., Badanes, Dmitrieva, & Watamura, 2012). This aspect of quality in the preschool classroom—teacher–child interactions and relationships—is the focus of this chapter, with an emphasis on links to children's activity in the HPA axis.

5.2 The HPA Axis in Early Childhood

The stress response system consists of three distinct structures—parasympathetic, sympathetic, and HPA axis (Del Giudice, Ellis, & Shirtclif, 2011). In response to a stressor, the parasympathetic and sympathetic systems are considered the first two responders, respectively, with need for activation building on the response of the previous system. If these systems are not able to successfully quell the stressor, the HPA axis provides a more consistent response through the release of cortisol that helps the individual return to homeostasis (Del Giudice et al., 2011; Gunnar & Quevedo, 2007). The HPA axis functions as a necessary and critical component of daily life, priming the individual to be vigilant through the release of the hormone cortisol (Gunnar & Quevedo, 2007). Typical patterns of cortisol follow a diurnal rhythm, with levels highest 30 min after wake and then a decline across the day with levels flattening in the evening and during sleep (Gunnar & Quevedo, 2007). Display of this rhythm is important as consistent deviations from this rise and fall (e.g., consistently showing high, flat levels of cortisol) are linked to consequences for children, such as higher levels of challenging behaviors (Alink et al., 2008; Shirtcliff, Granger, Booth, & Johnson, 2005).

5.2.1 *Relationships Shape the Developing HPA Axis*

The relationship a child has with his/her primary caregiver teaches the child appropriate strategies to regulate behaviors, emotions, stress, and cognition (Brownell & Kopp, 2007), and it plays a critical role in the development of the HPA axis in early childhood (Gunnar & Donzella, 2002; Meaney et al., 1996). Non-human experimental studies indicate that parent sensitivity and responsiveness have long-lasting effects on the stress response system (e.g., gene methylation, changes in ACTH and GC activity) and behavior (Levine, 2005). Children's attachment classification with their primary caregiver (usually their mother) has lasting effects on their behavior, relationships, and overall development. For example, children with a secure attachment are likely to display higher executive function skills in kindergarten (Bernier, Beauchamp, Carlson, & Lalonde, 2015), while children with an insecure or disorganized attachment are more likely to experience emotional or behavioral problems (van Ijzendoorn, Schuengel, & Bakersmans-Kranenburg, 1999). Similar patterns are evident with respect to activity in the HPA axis.

The relationship quality also matters for children's regulation of the HPA axis. For example, young children raised in neglected, deprived care are likely to display low levels of morning cortisol (for a review, see Gunnar & Vazquez, 2001). In response to a stressor, sensitive and responsive parenting affords children an increase in relational resources to utilize in the presence of a stressor— during a laboratory stressor, children who have a caregiver present with whom they have a secure attachment are less likely to experience a rise in cortisol (Nachmais, Gunnar, Mangelsdorf, Parritz, & Buss, 1996). On the other hand, a child with a disorganized attachment relationship is more likely to experience a longer activation of the HPA axis in response to the stressor (Hertsgaard, Gunnar, Erickson, & Nachmias, 1995). In addition to primary caregivers, children form relationships and attachment with other adults, including ECE teachers (Howes & Hamilton, 1992), who also plays a role in activity in the HPA axis.

5.2.2 Children's Cortisol in Early Care and Education Settings

Children often display cortisol levels that are higher at child care than in their home environment (Vermeer & van Ijzendoorn, 2006) although this dichotomy is not consistently supported in the research base (Vermeer et al., 2010). Regarding global and structural quality, there is mixed evidence supporting its role in affecting activity in children's HPA axis. Structural aspects of the classrooms, such as large group size, more adults, and smaller square footage are associated with higher levels of cortisol in preschool children (Legendre, 2003). Earlier work suggests mixed findings for global quality and children's cortisol with some indicating that children exhibit an increase in cortisol levels across the day regardless of quality (e.g., Dettling, Gunnar, & Donzella, 1999; Watamura, Donzella, Alwin, & Gunnar, 2003), and others indicating that children in mid-level global quality programs demonstrated a decline in cortisol levels across the day. Vermeer and van Ijzendoorn (2006) speculate that these mixed findings may be related to the general high-quality of these programs, thus limiting the variation of quality. Also, global quality, which captures structural and to some extent process quality features, may not lend itself to a critical, diverse lens of process quality given limited items to represent these features of classroom interactions.

Early work conducted by Dettling, Parker, Lane, Sebanc, and Gunnar (2000) found that children in classrooms with high levels of stimulation and learning displayed similar cortisol levels to home and demonstrated a decline across the day at child care. This is aligned with findings identifying structural quality as foundational, but that child outcomes, particularly language, are affected only when classroom interactions (process quality) are also of high quality (Mashburn et al., 2008). These initial findings are also well aligned with empirical work linking sensitive, responsive parent–child interactions to activity in the HPA axis. Since Dettling et al. (2000), research has expanded to examine relations between process quality and activity in the stress response system using more complex measurement and conceptualizations. The following section discusses two aspects of process quality: classroom relational quality and teacher–child relationship quality, and their associations with children's cortisol.

5.2.3 Classroom Relational Quality and Children's Cortisol

The emotional relational climate of the classroom, one marker of process quality, is linked to preschool children's cortisol levels (Hatfield et al., 2013; Sims, Guilfoyle, & Parry, 2006; Watamura, Kryzer, & Robertson, 2009). Relational climate in these three studies was observed across at least 1 day in the classroom, offering insight into the functioning of the classroom beyond teacher report. Cortisol samples were taken in the morning and afternoon for children over at least 2 days in all three studies.

Across these studies, the observational assessment of relational climate includes aspects of sensitivity, positive affect, and regard for the child using a variety of measures (Hatfield et al., 2013; Sims et al., 2006; Watamura et al., 2009). Classroom or teacher sensitivity is defined as ways in which the teacher listens and individually responds to each child, creating a warm and accepting atmosphere. Positive affect and warmth refers to ways in which teachers show affection and positive affect (e.g., smiling) in the classroom. And finally, regard captures ways in which teachers encourage children to express their ideas and be autonomous. These relational aspects of the classroom closely mirror relationship qualities in parent–child dyads that best support the HPA axis.

Results from these studies converge on the finding that children in classrooms rated high on these qualities are more likely to display more typical cortisol levels across the day at preschool. On the other hand, children in family child care programs that are more intrusive and rigid are likely to show an increase in cortisol across the day, in conflict with the expected decline (Gunnar, Kryzer, Van Ryzin, & Phillips, 2010); it should be noted that Gunnar et al. (2010) did not find an association with warm supportive classroom practices and children's cortisol in family child care homes. However, overall these findings suggest that in addition to the home microsystem playing a key role in children's developing HPA axis, the relational climate of the preschool classroom also demands attention.

In addition to classrooms that are high in sensitivity, positive affect, warmth, and support for children's autonomy, individual relationships with teachers play a role in children's developing HPA axis. Leveraging the research reviewed above on the importance of the relational climate in the classroom with the established research promoting teacher–child relationships and children's school readiness skills, an emerging research base identifying the role of individual teacher–child relationships on children's cortisol levels is discussed below.

5.2.4 Teacher–Child Relationships and Children's Cortisol

Children with close teacher–child relationships reap behavioral and academic benefits in early childhood and across the school years (Roorda et al., 2011). The developing evidence base for the role of teacher–child relationships on children's cortisol levels suggests that teacher–child closeness plays a role in children's cortisol levels at child care. Further, the specific pathways through which these relationships may support children are revealing a promising potential to protect children's activity in the HPA axis.

Badanes et al. (2012) examined links between teacher– and mother–child attachment styles and children's cortisol levels for 110 preschool children in 14 classrooms. While high security in the mother–child attachment played a positive role in children's cortisol patterns at child care, teacher–child relationships were also significant. Specifically, even after accounting for maternal security and host of child characteristics (e.g., temperament), teacher security predicted a decline in cortisol across the morning for children. This positive association is also evident in observations of teacher–child relationships. Children with a higher level of morning cortisol, compared to their classmates, were more likely to experience greater teacher sensitivity, a marker of a close teacher–child relationship, in the afternoon (Watamura et al., 2009).

Lisonbee et al. (2008) examined how close, dependent, and conflictual teacher–child relationships were related to children's cortisol. Children's cortisol levels and change within a setting (classroom and play task) were examined. Children whose teachers rated them as clingier (e.g., the child often asks for help even if he/she does not need it) were more likely to display higher afternoon cortisol levels and demonstrate an increase in cortisol across the day even after accounting for a host of covariates. Significant, bivariate correlations emerged for teacher–child closeness and children's cortisol change during the teacher–child play task such that those with closer relationships demonstrated a decline in cortisol during the task. The opposite was found for children with high conflict in the relationship as those children displayed an increase across the task.

5.2.4.1 Banking Time

Given the abundance of research demonstrating the positive affect that teacher–child closeness has on children's academics, behaviors, and biology, it is unsurprising that there are a variety of classroom- and teacher-focused interventions aimed at increasing the quality of teacher–child relationships. One such intervention for preschool-age children, *Banking Time* (Pianta & Hamre, 2001) has shown effectiveness across three separate studies. *Banking Time* is built on attachment theory, arguing that children need a sensitive, responsive caregiver in order to fully engage, and feel supported, in the learning environment. The teacher is asked to spend one-on-one time with the child two to three times a week for 7 weeks, allowing the child to lead the play. These sessions are videorecorded and the teacher is encouraged to use strategies such as observation, narration, and labeling (e.g., emotions) and meet with a consultant biweekly. The hope is that teachers learn through video review with their consultant how to respond warmly, with acceptance, and with high regard for the child in order to build a close relationship (Pianta & Hamre, 2001).

Beyond a correlational study that demonstrated positive associations between teacher's use of *Banking Time* and teacher–child closeness (Driscoll, Wang, Mashburn, & Pianta, 2011), two experimental studies also tout the benefits of this intervention. First, a small-scale intervention study demonstrated meaningful differences in the experimental group via increased teacher–child closeness and decreases in children's disruptive behavior in the classroom compared to the control group (Driscoll & Pianta, 2010). Recently, a large randomized control trial ($n = 470$ preschool children, 183 teachers) reported positive changes in observed teacher behavior as well as lower levels of children's externalizing behaviors (Williford et al., 2017) for children with disruptive behaviors. This explicit focus on children with disruptive behaviors afforded an opportunity to examine the effectiveness of this intervention for children who were already at risk for abberant cortisol patterns (Alink et al., 2008). Within Williford et al. (2017), a subsample of these children ($n = 113$ children, 70 teachers) also provided saliva samples that were assayed for cortisol.

Hatfield and Williford (2017) examined changes in preschool children's cortisol levels at child care for a subset of 113 children with disruptive behaviors. Change in cortisol across the morning at school was measured in winter and at the end of the school year. In winter, children's cortisol levels did not differ between the intervention groups. However, at the end of the school year, children whose teachers participated in *Banking Time,* compared to the control group, displayed a decline in cortisol across the morning. The control group displayed an increase in cortisol across the morning at child care. The results from this quasi-experimental study suggest that investing in teacher–child relationships may have the potential to change children's functioning in the HPA axis. Similar relationship-driven interventions with children and families in foster care also support positive change in children's cortisol levels (Dozier, Peloso, Lewis, Laurenceau, & Levine, 2008; Fisher, Gunnar, Chamberlain, & Reid, 2000).

Over a decade ago, a meta-analysis reported that children displayed higher levels of cortisol at child care compared to home (Vermeer & van Ijzendoorn, 2006), spurring research that aimed to identify the classroom and relational conditions under which children experience a rise in cortisol at child care. Aspects of process quality, specifically the positive relational classroom climate and close teacher–child relationships, seem to protect children from the rise in cortisol at child care. Recent work also points to the success of a teacher-focused relationship intervention,

Banking Time, on changing children's cortisol patterns. The evidence indicates that relationships within ECE settings, particularly in preschool classrooms, warrant attention from stakeholders, the ECE workforce, and families.

5.3 Implications

It is clear that relationships children have with adults play a role in the development of children's HPA axis and school readiness skills. Correlational evidence indicates that responsive caregiving buffers the negative consequences of being reared in a deprived environment (Loman et al., 2010) and that children with a secure attachment are better able to cope with a stressor (Nachmais et al., 1996). Animal experimental models confirm these pathways between relationships and the HPA axis (Meaney et al., 1996). Finally, emerging experimental evidence from a variety of disciplines (i.e., education, social work) demonstrates the positive effect that sensitive adult–child relationships have on children's cortisol levels (Dozier et al., 2008; Fisher et al., 2000; Hatfield & Williford, 2017). Given this evidence, it is critical that state and national early education systems reflect the importance of relationships in standards, which should also inform professional development for the ECE workforce. Further, families need to be aware of the importance of ECE environments and ways to advocate for quality ECE programming.

5.3.1 Implications for Practice and/or Policy

Within this decade, ECE systems are, to some extent, assessing the relational climate of the classroom in national and state standards or ratings with the Classroom Assessment Scoring System (CLASS) Pre-k; Pianta, La Paro, & Hamre, 2008). The CLASS Pre-k, a measure of process quality, includes a domain of Emotional Support, which assesses the relational climate (e.g., teacher sensitivity, positive climate). The Office of Head Start mandated that all grantees receive a rating on the CLASS as part of redesignation, recognizing the importance of these types of teacher–child interactions. Currently, 22 states or districts use the CLASS in their quality rating and improvement system (QRIS) to rate the quality of ECE programs (Teachstone, 2016). Other states rate quality within their QRIS system, but utilize a measure of global quality (e.g., Environmental Rating Scales) or a self-developed tool. Whatever the assessment tool, systems should also focus on the relationships and interactions children have with adults in their ECE setting.

Another support that deserves attention is preservice training and inservice professional development opportunities for ECE teachers that are focused on these types of interactions and relationships. For preservice teachers, video review and reflective practice that is embedded in course work and practicum demonstrate promise in changing teaching practices. In university courses, a CLASS-focused video review of an individual's teaching practice demonstrates mixed findings for teaching quality. Some evidence indicates no change in practice, with respect to classroom management and instructional behaviors and a decline in responsivity (La Paro, Maynard, Thomason, & Scott-Little, 2012). A different study led teachers to think more critically about their skills, identify weaknesses, and identify opportunities for teachable moments (Bayat, 2010). At a larger scale, the University of Washington has partnered with the Office of Head Start to create the EarlyEdU Alliance™, a suite of courses and materials for higher education programs focused on effective teacher–child interactions, with the aim to increase attainment of Bachelor's degrees for the ECE workforce (EarlyEDU Alliance™, 2016).

For inservice teachers, effective professional development opportunities are often in the form of interventions, and are more time and effort intensive. As previously reviewed, *Banking Time*, shows positive effects on teaching practices, relationships, child behavior, and children's activity in the stress response system (Driscoll & Pianta, 2010; Hatfield & Williford, 2017; Williford et al., 2017), however, the program is very time intensive. Other coaching interventions focused on responsive teacher–child interactions and/or building close teacher–child relationships with preschool children, such as My Teaching Partner (MTP), show promise in changing practice and child behavior, but are also time intensive. Although intensive, components of MTP and MTP-like programs are scalable. Georgia recently piloted two CLASS-based professional development programs that were modified from the original forms: MTP (Georgia teachers completed an average of eight cycles) and Making the Most of Classroom Interactions (MMCI); a peer cohort model with 5 full-day workshops. Results from a 3-year study with 486 teachers show that MMCI and MTP are effective in increasing classroom practice; however, only MMCI showed improvements in more than one CLASS domain (Early, Maxwell, Ponder, & Pan, 2017). Scalable efforts like these in Georgia and others (e.g., Head Start CARES project) show promise in scaling these effective intervention programs thereby increasing ECE professionals' knowledge and skills in responsive teaching.

5.3.2 *Implications for Understanding Family Resilience*

Families serve as the principal influence on children (National Academics of Sciences, Engineering, & Medicine, 2016), and the parent–child relationship is a key factor in promoting resilience, particularly with the stress response system (Zalewski, Lengua, Kiff, & Fisher, 2012). With respect to children's stress response system, the role of the mother–child relationship is important to consider within the ECE classroom. This is represented in the early work suggesting that children do not show a rise in cortisol at home, but only show a rise in the ECE setting (see Vermeer & van Ijzendoorn, 2006 for a review). Additionally, the mother–child relationship interacts with child care quality to affect children's cortisol in positive and negative ways. Results from Badanes et al. (2012) indicate that children with a secure attachment with their mother, but enrolled in classrooms of lower quality, display increasing cortisol patterns across the day, but those with a less secure attachment to their mother demonstrate a flat pattern of activity regardless of ECE quality. However, when children experience double protection—high quality in both the mother–child relationship and classroom environment, they are more likely to show a decline in cortisol across the day (Badanes et al., 2012). Child care can also exacerbate negative consequences for children's HPA axis for children with a poor mother–child relationship. Maternal insensitivity and time in child care at age three uniquely predict lower awakening cortisol at age 15 (Roisman et al., 2009).

There are a few ways to promote resilience in families and young children given this evidence. First, families should identify quality child care programs with the help of state systems like QRIS or enrolling their child in a Head Start program given that ECE quality matters for promoting a healthy stress response system in young children. State systems should improve visibility of their QRIS so that parents are aware of this resource; a report from Child Trends (Walter, Torres, & Aldebot-Green, 2015) offers some suggestions for this. Second, families should aim to create positive relationships with the ECE teachers who care for their child(ren). Family involvement in school, even in preschool, can have spillover effects into the family unit. For example, parents who were more involved with their child's Head Start program were more likely to report higher quality home interactions (e.g., taught child letters) and less spanking in the home at the end of the year (Ansari & Gershoff, 2016). Finally, investment in parenting education programs to promote positive parenting are effective in promoting positive parenting practices, such as sensitive, responsive parenting (Menting, Orobio de Castro, & Matthys, 2013).

5.4 Conclusion and Future Directions

5.4.1 Summary of Main Discussion Points

The HPA axis is malleable in early childhood and sensitive to environmental inputs, especially relationships with primary caregivers, including ECE teachers. The likelihood preschool children experience a program with high-quality teacher–child relationships is low (Hamre, 2014), which is concerning given that the majority of preschool-aged children are enrolled in some type of ECE program. The benefits of high-quality preschool programming are overwhelming with respect to children's school readiness skills (Phillips et al., 2017), family well-being (Press et al., 2006), and financial investments (Reynolds & Temple, 2008), and the research concerning high-quality preschool and children's activity in the HPA axis are encouraging. Numerous studies indicate that the interactions children experience in preschool affect their cortisol levels, such that sensitive, responsive interactions promote a typical decline in cortisol across the day (e.g., Sims et al., 2006). Further, a quasi-experimental study found that children whose teacher participated in a relationship-building focused intervention had a decline in cortisol across the morning, compared to children in the control group (Hatfield & Williford, 2017). This echoes intervention results from other disciplines (e.g., Dozier et al., 2008), and initially suggests implications for policy, practices, and families.

5.4.2 *Limitations*

While it is beyond the scope of this chapter to discuss all factors that contribute to children's developing HPA axis and cortisol levels, some additional family-, child-, and classroom-level factors are discussed. Within the family, income is linked to more aberrant cortisol patterns even after accounting for the parent–child relationship (Zalewski, Lengua, Thompson, & Kiff, 2016). Family conflict also influences cortisol responses for preschool children (Robles, Chap. 8, this volume; Slatcher & Robles, 2012). Child behavior (e.g., hyperactivity, aggression) also plays a role in children's stress response system. Preschool-aged children with externalizing behaviors are more likely to display higher cortisol levels (Alink et al., 2008), but gender and temperament may contribute to this association (Dettling et al., 1999; Gunnar et al., 2010).

Regarding the ECE setting, other factors in addition to quality should be understood. For instance, dosage of child care is an important factor, as a recent study found that full-day preschool was detrimental to children's cortisol patterns on home-care and child-care day (Lumian, Dmitrieva, Mendoza, Badanes, & Watamura, 2016). Other studies have also reported that previous experience in child care contributes to children's cortisol levels in child care (Ouellet-Morin et al., 2010). Importantly, there is emerging evidence that higher dosage may be protective (leads to lower cortisol levels) for children from high-risk families, but not those from low-risk families (Berry, Blair, Granger, & The Family Life Project Key Investigators, 2016). Finally, there is a need to extend the setting from center-based care into home-based child care (e.g., family child care homes, family-, friend-, and neighbor care) in the United States (see Gunnar et al., 2010 for an exception) to better understand associations with children's cortisol levels, as evidence suggests differences by type of care for quality (Bassok, Fitzpatrick, Greenberg, & Loeb, 2016).

5.4.3 *Future Directions*

Future research should investigate longitudinal associations, examine the role of peers in the classroom, and identify specific behavioral strategies for teachers and children. Longitudinal analyses should extend from early childhood to school-aged children in order to identify the factors that continually support children's HPA axis. In infancy and toddlerhood, child care attendance is linked to higher cortisol patterns (Ahnert, Gunnar, Lamb, & Barthel, 2004; Ouellet-Morin et al., 2010). In preschool (Hatfield et al., 2013) to first grade (Ahnert, Harwardt-Heinecke,

Kappler, Eckstein-Madry, & Milatz, 2012), relationships children have with teachers play a protective role in that these children are more likely to show a decline in cortisol across the day at school. However, the long-term benefits of these teacher–child relationships are unknown. Relatedly, a child's classroom experience and school readiness skills are affected by the peers in the classroom (e.g., Mashburn, Justice, Downer, & Pianta, 2009; Yudron, Jones, & Raver, 2014), and it is likely that the HPA axis is also affected by classroom composition. For example, Berry et al. (2016) found that toddlers with greater exposure to peers in ECE settings were more likely to have lower cortisol levels at home, and Watamura et al. (2013) found that toddlers who engaged in more play with peers had lower cortisol levels at child care. It is likely that quality of these interactions and relationships also play a critical role in understanding the mechanisms between peers and preschool children's cortisol levels.

There is robust evidence that early relationships, including those in ECE settings, affect children's school readiness skills, and emerging evidence supporting its role in preschool children's HPA axis. In addition to the above, research must move to identifying scalable supports for families and ECE professionals in order to best support young children. Promising early childhood programs and curriculum that focus on supporting children's self-regulatory skills (i.e., Tools of the Mind, Kids in Transition to School) are also demonstrating positive associations with children's salivary cortisol levels and other school readiness skills (Blair & Raver, 2014; Pears, Graham, Kim, & Fisher, 2013). Focusing on building relationships and supporting positive behavior regulation skills for young children seem to be the levers for change within ECE programming. Through identification of the critical components of effective interventions and programs, we can uncover how to best, and efficiently, support the health and well-being of young children.

Questions for Thought and Discussion

1. What role do relationships with parents play in the development of the HPA axis?
2. Describe how process quality, particularly relational climate and teacher–child interactions, are associated with children's cortisol levels.
3. How might children's experiences in the classroom vary by child characteristics such as self-regulation skills? Can you think of scenarios in which a child's self-regulation skills may play a key role in the regulation of his/her stress response system?
4. Thinking about responsive teacher–child interactions and their relation to children's HPA axis, how might you coach a teacher to respond in the following scenario?

   Ms. Brice has been very frustrated with Jill these past few days. Jill has been pushing her friends on the playground and unable to focus on her table work. During dramatic play, Jill reaches over and grabs a bowl from a peer, Ms. Brice yells, "Jill, stop it! Why can't you just play well with your friends! What is wrong with you?"

5. What may be some challenges to scalability of interventions that are time and resource intensive, like *Banking Time*? Can you identify some solutions to these challenges to scalability?
6. While aberrant cortisol levels lead to negative outcomes for children, individuals need activation of their stress response system to learn to cope with stressors and manage daily life. Discuss two scenarios considering socioemotional and then cognitive skills, in which activation in the stress response system would be positive for preschool children. What do those scenarios look like?
7. Peer composition, or classroom composition effects, are becoming important to consider in a variety of child outcomes. This chapter speculates the importance of peers and there is limited research to suggest peers are important when it comes to children's activity in the stress response system. Expand on this and give your own ideas as to what role peers play.

Glossary

Classroom relational climate A construct of classroom process quality that focuses explicitly on responsive, warm, and sensitive teacher–child interactions at the classroom level.

Close teacher–child relationship A teacher–child relationship that is characterizied by sensitive and warm interactions, children's use of the teacher as a secure base, and display of positive affection.

Cortisol A hormone produced by the HPA axis that affords the ability to cope with stressors and daily life. Cortisol is expected to be the highest approximately 30 min after wake and then decline across the day.

Early care and education A setting (e.g., center, family child care home) that serves children 0–5 years. The focus of these settings is on the care, education, and development of young children.

Hypothalamic pituitary adrenal (HPA) axis HPA axis provides a more consistent response (compared to the sympathetic and parasympathetic systems) through the release of cortisol that helps the individual return to homeostasis. It primes the individual to be vigilant through the release of the hormone cortisol.

Process quality A construct of classroom quality that focuses on relationships and interactions between teachers and children and among peers.

School readiness A set of skills which include cognitive (e.g., language), social (e.g., peer relations), emotional (e.g., regulation of anger), and behavioral (e.g., impulse control) competencies that children should possess to be ready for school. Often refered to as skills children need to be ready for kindergarten/formal schooling.

Secure attachment An attachment classification coined by Mary Ainsworth that characterizes an adult–child relationship that is sensitive, warm, and responsive. In a secure adult–child attachment, the child uses the adult as a secure base.

Stress response system Comprised of three distinct structures—parasympathetic, sympathetic, and hypothalamic pituitary adrenal (HPA) axis that react in response to a stressor.

Structural quality A construct of classroom quality that focuses on largely physical factors such as teacher education level, curriculum, ratio, and classroom materials.

References

Ahnert, L., Gunnar, M. G., Lamb, M. E., & Barthel, M. (2004). Transition to child care: Associations with infant-mother attachment, infant negative emotion, and cortisol elevations. *Child Development, 75*, 639–650. https://doi.org/10.1111/j.1467-8624.2004.00698.x

Ahnert, L., Harwardt-Heinecke, E., Kappler, G., Eckstein-Madry, T., & Milatz, A. (2012). Student-teacher relationships and classroom climate in first grade: How do they relate to students' stress regulation? *Attachment & Human Development, 14*, 249–263. https://doi.org/10.1080/14616734.2012.673277

Alink, L. R. A., van Ijzendoorn, M. H., Bakermans-Kranenburg, M. J., Mesman, J., Juffer, F., & Koot, H. M. (2008). Cortisol and externalizing behavior in children and adolescents: Mixed meta-analytic evidence for the inverse relation of basal cortisol and cortisol reactivity with externalizing behavior. *Developmental Psychobiology, 50*, 427–450. https://doi.org/10.1002/dev.20300

Ansari, A., & Gershoff, E. (2016). Parent involvement in Head Start and children's development: Indirect effects through parenting. *Journal of Marriage and Family, 78*, 562–579. https://doi.org/10.1111/jomf.12266

Badanes, L. S., Dmitrieva, J., & Watamura, S. E. (2012). Understanding cortisol reactivity across the day at child care: The potential buffering role of secure attachments to caregivers. *Early Childhood Research Quarterly, 27*, 156–165. https://doi.org/10.1016/j.ecresq.2011.05.005

Bassok, D., Fitzpatrick, M., Greenberg, E., & Loeb, S. (2016). Within- and between-sector quality differences in early childhood education and care. *Child Development, 87*, 1627–1645. https://doi.org/10.1111/cdev.12551

Bayat, M. (2010). Use of dialogue journals and video-recording in early childhood teacher education. *Journal of Early Childhood Teacher Education, 31*, 159–172. https://doi.org/10.1080/10901021003781247

Bernier, A., Beauchamp, M. H., Carlson, S. M., & Lalonde, G. (2015) A secure base from which to regulate: Attachment security in toddlerhood as a predictor of executive functioning at school entry. *Developmental Psychology, 51*, 1177–1189. https://doi.org/10.1037/dev0000032

Bernier, A., Carlson, S. M., & Whipple, N. (2010). From external regulation to self-regulation: Early parenting precursors of young children's executivefunctioning. *Child Development, 81*, 326–339. https://doi.org/10.1111/j.1467-8624.2009.01397.x

Berry, D., Blair, C., Granger, D. A., & The Family Life Project Key Investigators. (2016). Child care and cortisol across infancy and toddlerhood: Poverty, peers, and developmental timing. *Family Relations, 65*, 51–72. https://doi.org/10.1111/fare.12184

Birch, S. H., & Ladd, G. W. (1997). The teacher-child relationship and children's early school adjustment. *Journal of School Psychology, 35*, 61–79. https://doi.org/10.1016/S0022-4405(96)00029-5

Blair, C., & Raver, C. C. (2014). Closing the achievement gap through modification of neurocognitive and neuroendocrine function: Results from a cluster randomized controlled trial of an innovative approach to the education of children in lindergarten. *PLoS One, 9*(11), e112393. https://doi.org/10.1371/journal.pone.0112393

Bronfenbrenner, U., & Morris, P. A. (2006). The bioecological model of human development. In W. Damon, & R. M. Lerner (Eds.), *Handbook of child psychology* (Vol. 1: Theoretical models of human development, 6th ed., pp. 793–828). Hoboken, NJ: Wiley.

Brownell, C. A., & Kopp, C. B. (Eds.). (2007). *Socioemotional development in the toddler years: Transitions and transformations*. New York, NY: Guilford.

Burchinal, M., Howes, C., Pianta, R., Bryant, D., Early, D., Clifford, R., & Barbarin, O. (2008). Predicting child outcomes at the end of kindergarten from the quality of pre-kindergarten teacher–child interactions and instruction. *Applied Developmental Science, 12*, 140–153. https://doi.org/10.1080/10888690802199418

Burchinal, M., Vandergift, N., Pianta, R., & Mashburn, A. (2010). Threshold analysis of association between child care quality and child outcomes for low-income children in pre-kindergarten programs. *Early Childhood Research Quarterly, 25*, 166–176. https://doi.org/10.1016/j.ecresq.2009.10.004

Burchinal, M. R., Roberts, J. E., Riggins, R., Jr., Zeisel, S. A., Neebe, E., & Bryant, D. (2000). Relating quality of center-based child care to early cognitive and language development longitudinally. *Child Development, 71*, 339–357. https://doi.org/10.1111/1467-8624.00149

Campbell, F., Conti, G., Heckman, J. J., Moon, S. H., Pinto, R., Pungello, E., & Pan, Y. (2014). Early childhood investments substantially boost adult health. *Science, 343*, 1478–1485. https://doi.org/10.1126/science

Danziger, S. K., Ananat, E. O., & Browning, K. G. (2004). Childcare subsidies and the transition from welfare to work. *Family Relations, 53*, 219–228. https://doi.org/10.1111/j.0022-2445.2004.00012.x

Del Giudice, M., Ellis, B. J., & Shirtclif, E. A. (2011). The adaptive calibration model of stress responsivity. *Neuroscience and Biobehavioral Reviews, 35*, 1562–1592. https://doi.org/10.1016/j.neubiorev.2010.11.007

Dettling, A. C., Gunnar, M. R., & Donzella, B. (1999). Cortisol levels of young children in full-day childcare centers: Relations with age and temperament. *Psychoneuroendocrinology, 24*, 519–536. https://doi.org/10.1016/S0306-4530(99)00009-8

Dettling, A. C., Parker, S. W., Lane, S., Sebanc, A., & Gunnar, M. R. (2000). Quality of care and temperament determine changes in cortisol concentrations over the day for young children in childcare. *Psychoneuroendocrinology, 25*, 819–836. https://doi.org/10.1016/S0306-4530(00)00028-7

Dozier, M., Peloso, E., Lewis, E., Laurenceau, J. P., & Levine, S. (2008). Effects of an attachment-based intervention on the cortisol production of infants and toddlers in foster care. *Development and Psychopathology, 20*, 845–859. https://doi.org/10.1017/S0954579408000400

Driscoll, K., & Pianta, R. (2010). Banking time in Head Start: Early efficacy of an intervention designed to promote supportive teacher-child relationships. *Early Education and Development, 21*, 38–64. https://doi.org/10.1080/10409280802657449

Driscoll, K. C., Wang, L., Mashburn, A. J., & Pianta, R. C. (2011). Fostering supportive teacher-child relationships: Intervention implementation in a state-funded preschool program. *Early Education and Development, 22*, 593–619. https://doi.org/10.1080/10409289.2010.502015

Early, D. M., Maxwell, K. L., Ponder, B. D., & Pan, Y. (2017). Improving teacher-child interactions: A randomized controlled trial of Making the Most of Classroom Interactions and My Teaching Partner professional development models. *Early Childhood Research Quarterly, 38*, 57–70. https://doi.org/10.1016/j.ecresq.2016.08.005

EarlyEdU Alliance™. (2016). *Early EdU - An alliance of Head Start and early learning*. Retrieved from http://www.earlyedualliance.org/.

Fisher, P. A., Gunnar, M. R., Chamberlain, P., & Reid, J. B. (2000). Preventive intervention for maltreated preschool children: Impact on children's behavior, neuroendocrine activity, and foster parent functioning. *Journal of the American Academy of Child & Adolescent Psychiatry, 39*, 1356–1364. https://doi.org/10.1097/00004583-200011000-00009

Gelber, A., & Isen, A. (2013). Children's schooling and parents' behavior: Evidence from the Head Start impact study. *Journal of Public Economics, 101*, 35–38. https://doi.org/10.1016/j.jpubeco.2013.02.005

Gunnar, M., & Quevedo, K. (2007). The neurobiology of stress and development. *Annual Review of Psychology, 58*, 145–173. https://doi.org/10.1146/annurev.psych.58.110405.085605

Gunnar, M. R., & Donzella, B. (2002). Social regulation of the cortisol levels in early human development. *Psychoneuroendocrinology, 27*, 199–220. https://doi.org/10.1016/S0306-4530(01)00045-2

Gunnar, M. R., Kryzer, E., Van Ryzin, M. J., & Phillips, D. A. (2010). The rise in cortisol in family day care: Associations with aspects of care quality, child behavior, and child sex. *Child Development, 81*, 851–869. https://doi.org/10.1111/j.1467-8624.2010.01438.x

Gunnar, M. R., & Vazquez, D. M. (2001). Low cortisol and a flattening of expected daytime rhythm: Potential indices of risk in human development. *Development and Psychopathology, 13*, 515–538. https://doi.org/10.1017/s0954579401003066

Hamre, B. K. (2014). Teachers' daily interactions with children: An essential ingredient in effective early childhood programs. *Child Development Perspectives, 8*, 223–230. https://doi.org/10.1111/cdep.12090

Hamre, B. K., Hatfield, B. E., Pianta, R. C., & Jamil, F. (2014). Evidence for general and domain specific elements of teacher-child interactions: Associations with preschool children's development. *Child Development, 85*, 1257–1274. https://doi.org/10.1111/cdev.12184

Hatfield, B. E., Burchinal, M. R., Pianta, R. C., & Sideris, J. (2016). Thresholds in the association between quality of teacher-child interactions and preschool children's school readiness skills. *Early Childhood Research Quarterly, 36*, 561–571. https://doi.org/10.1016/j.ecresq.2015.09.005

Hatfield, B. E., Hestenes, L. L., Kintner-Duffy, V. L., & O'Brien, M. (2013). Classroom emotional support predicts differences in preschool children's cortisol and alpha-amylase levels. *Early Childhood Research Quarterly, 28*, 347–356. https://doi.org/10.1016/j.ecresq.2012.08.001

Hatfield, B. E., & Williford, A. P. (2017). Cortisol patterns for young children displaying disruptive behavior: Effects linked to a teacher-child, relationship-focused intervention. *Prevention Science, 18*, 40–49. https://doi.org/10.1007/s11121-016-0693-9

Hertsgaard, L., Gunnar, M., Erickson, M. F., & Nachmias, M. (1995). Adrenocortical responses to the strange situation in infants with disorganized/disoriented attachment relationships. *Child Development, 66*, 1100–1106. https://doi.org/10.1111/j.1467-8624.1995.tb00925.x

Hestenes, L., Cassidy, D., Hegde, A., & Lower, J. K. (2007). Quality in inclusive and non-inclusive infant and toddler classrooms. *Journal of Research in Childhood Education, 22*, 69–84. https://doi.org/10.1080/02568540709594613

Hirsh-Pasek, K., Adamson, L. B., Bakeman, R., Owen, M. T., Golinkoff, R. M., Pace, A., … Suma, K. (2015). The contribution of early communication quality to low-income children's language success. *Psychological Science, 26*, 1071–1083. https://doi.org/10.1177/0956797615581493

Howes, C. (2000). Social-emotional classroom climate in child care, child–teacher relationships and children's second grade peer relations. *Social Development, 9*, 191–204. https://doi.org/10.1111/1467-9507.00119

Howes, C., & Hamilton, C. E. (1992). Children's relationships with caregivers: Mothers and child care teachers. *Child Development, 63*, 859–866.. Retrieved from http://www.jstor.org/stable/1131238

La Paro, K. M., Maynard, C., Thomason, A., & Scott-Little, C. (2012). Developing teachers' classroom interactions: A description of a video review process for early childhood education students. *Journal of Early Childhood Teacher Education, 33*, 224–238. https://doi.org/10.1080/10901027.2012.705809

Laughlin, L. (2013). *Who's minding the kids? Child care arrangements: Spring 2011*. Retrieved from http://www.census.gov/library/publications/2013/demo/p70-135.html.

Legendre, A. (2003). Environmental features influencing toddlers' bioemotional reactions in day care centers. *Environment and Behavior, 35*, 523–548. https://doi.org/10.1177/0013916503035004005

Levine, S. (2005). Developmental determinants of sensitivity and resistance to stress. *Psychoneuoendocrinology, 30*, 939–946. https://doi.org/10.1016/j.psyneuen.2005.03.013

Lisonbee, J. A., Mize, J., Lapp Payne, A., & Granger, D. A. (2008). Children's cortisol and the quality of teacher–child relationships in child care. *Child Development, 79*, 1818–1832. https://doi.org/10.1111/j.1467-8624.2008.01228.x

Loman, M. M., Gunnar, M. R., & The Early Experience, Stress, & Neurobehavioral Development Center. (2010). Early experience and the development of stress reactivity and regulation in children. *Neuroscience & Biobehavioral Reviews, 34*, 867–876. https://doi.org/10.1016/j.neubiorev.2009.05.007

Ludwig, J., & Miller, D. L. (2007). Does Head Start improve children's life chances? Evidence from a regression discontinuity design. *The Quarterly Journal of Economics, 122*, 159–208. https://doi.org/10.1162/qjec.122.1.159.z

Lumian, D. S., Dmitrieva, J., Mendoza, M. M., Badanes, L. S., & Watamura, S. E. (2016). The impact of program structure on cortisol patterning in children attending out-of-home child care. *Early Childhood Research Quarterly, 34*, 92–103. https://doi.org/10.1016/j.ecresq.2015.09.004

Marshall, N. L., Wagner Robeson, W., Tracy, A. J., Frye, A., & Roberts, J. (2013). Subsidized child care, maternal employment and access to quality, affordable child care. *Early Childhood Research Quarterly, 28*, 808–819. https://doi.org/10.1016/j.ecresq.2013.07.008

Mashburn, A. J., Downer, J. T., Hamre, B. K., Justice, L. M., & Pianta, R. C. (2010). Consultation for teachers and children's language and literacy development during pre-kindergarten. *Applied Developmental Science, 14*, 179–196. https://doi.org/10.1080/10888691.2010.516187

Mashburn, A. J., Justice, L. M., Downer, J. T., & Pianta, R. C. (2009). Peer effects on children's language achievement during pre-kindergarten. *Child Development, 80*, 686–702. https://doi.org/10.1111/j.1467-8624.2009.01291.x

Mashburn, A. J., Pianta, R. C., Hamre, B. K., Downer, J. T., Barbarin, O. A., Bryant, D., … Howes, C. (2008). Measures of classroom quality in prekindergarten and children's development of academic, language, and social skills. *Child Development, 79*, 732–749. https://doi.org/10.1111/j.1467-8624.2008.01154.x

Meaney, M. J. (2001). Maternal care, gene expression, and the transmission of individual differences in stress reactivity across generations. *Annual Review of Neuroscience, 24*, 1161–1192. https://doi.org/10.1146/annurev.neuro.24.1.1161

Meaney, M. J., Diorio, J., Francis, D., Widdowson, J., La Plante, P., Caldji, C., … Plotsky, P. M. (1996). Early environmental regulation of forebrain glucocorticoids receptor gene expression: Implications for adrenocortical responses to stress. *Developmental Neuroscience, 18*, 49–60. https://doi.org/10.1159/000111396

Menting, A. T. A., Orobio de Castro, B., & Matthys, W. (2013). Effectiveness of the incredible years parent training to modify disruptive and prosocial child behavior: A meta-analytic review. *Clinical Psychology Review, 33*, 901–913. https://doi.org/10.1016/j.cpr.2013.07.006

Nachmais, M., Gunnar, M. R., Mangelsdorf, S., Parritz, R. H., & Buss, K. (1996). Behavioral inhibition and stress reactivity: The moderating role of attachment security. *Child Development, 67*, 508–522. https://doi.org/10.1111/j.1467-8624.1996.tb01748.x

National Academics of Sciences, Engineering, & Medicine. (2016). *Parenting matters: Supporting parents of children ages* (pp. 0–8). Washington, DC: The National Academies Press.

Ouellet-Morin, I., Tremblay, R. E., Boivin, M., Meaney, M., Kramer, M., & Côté, S. M. (2010). Diurnal cortisol secretion at home and in child care: A prospective study of 2-year-old toddlers. *Journal of Child Psychology and Psychiatry, 51*, 295–303. https://doi.org/10.1111/j.1469-7610.2009.02167.x

Pears, K. C., Graham, A. M., Kim, H. L., & Fisher, P. A. (2013, April). *Effects of a school readiness intervention for children in foster care on diurnal cortisol at the start of school.* Paper presented at the Society for Research in Child Development, Seattle, WA.

Phillips, D. A., Lipsey, M. W., Dodge, K. A., Haskins, R., Bassok, D., Burchinal, M. R., … Weiland, C. (2017). *Puzzling it out: The current state of scientific knowledge on pre-kindergarten effects: A consensus statement.* Retrieved from https://www.brookings.edu/wp-content/uploads/2017/04/consensus-statement_final.pdf.

Pianta, R. C., & Hamre, B. K. (2001). *Banking time: Pre-K manual.* Charlottesville, VA: The Center for Advanced Study of Teaching and Learning at the University of Virginia. Retrieved from http://www.lookconsultation.org/resources/BankingTime-Resource1.pdf

Pratt, M., Lipscomb, S. T., & Schmitt, S. A. (2015). The effect of Head Start on parenting outcomes for children living in non-parental care. *Journal of Child and Family Studies, 24*, 2944–2956. https://doi.org/10.1007/s10826-014-0098-y

Press, J. E., Fagan, J., & Laughlin, L. (2006). Taking pressure off families: Child-care subsidies lessen mothers' work-hour problems. *Journal of Marriage and Family, 68*, 155–171. https://doi.org/10.1111/j.1741-3737.2006.00240.x

Pianta, R. C., La Paro, K. M., & Hamre, B. K. (2008). *Classroom Assessment Scoring System [CLASS] manual: Pre-k*. Baltimore, MD: Paul H. Brookes.

Reynolds, A. J., & Temple, J. A. (2008). Cost-effective early childhood development programs from preschool to third grade. *Annual Review of Clinical Psychology, 4*, 109–139. https://doi.org/10.1146/annurev.clinpsy.3.022806.091411

Roisman, G. I., Susman, E., Barnett-Walker, K., Booth-LaForce, C., Owen, M. T., Belsky, J., … The NICHD Early Child Care Research Network. (2009). Early family and child-care antecedents of awakening cortisol levels in adolescence. *Child Development, 80*, 907–920. https://doi.org/10.1111/j.1467-8624.2009.01305.x

Romano, E., Kohen, D., & Findlay, L. C. (2010). Associations among child care, family, and behavior outcomes in a nation-wide sample of preschool-aged children. *International Journal of Behavioral Development, 34*, 427–440. https://doi.org/10.1177/0165025409351657

Roorda, D. L., Koomen, H. M. Y., Split, J. L., & Oort, F. J. (2011). The influence of affective teacher-student relationships on students' school engagement and achievement: A meta-analytic approach. *Review of Educational Research, 81*, 493–529. https://doi.org/10.3102/0034654311421793

Sabol, T. J., & Hoyt, L. T. (2017). The long arm of childhood: Preschool associations with adolescent health. *Developmental Psychology, 53*, 752–763. https://doi.org/10.1037/dev0000287

Sajaniemi, N., Suhonen, E., Hotulainen, R., Tormanen, M., Alijoki, A., Nislin, M., & Kontu, K. (2011). Demographic factors, temperament and the quality of the preschool environment as predictors of daily cortisol changes among Finnish six-year-old children. *European Early Childhood Education Research Journal, 22*, 286–306. https://doi.org/10.1080/1350293X.2013.783303

Schmidt, M. B., Pentimonti, J. M., & Justice, L. M. (2012). Teacher-child relationships, behavior regulation, and language gain among at-risk preschoolers. *Journal of School Psychology, 50*, 681–699. https://doi.org/10.1016/j.jsp.2012.04.003

Schober, P. S., & Spiess, C. K. (2015). Local day care quality and maternal employment: Evidence From East and West Germany. *Family Relations, 77*, 712–729. https://doi.org/10.1111/jomf.12180

Shirtcliff, E. A., Granger, D. A., Booth, A., & Johnson, D. (2005). Low salivary cortisol levels and externalizing behavior problems in youth. *Development and Pathology, 17*, 167–184. https://doi.org/10.1017/S095457940505009

Silver, R. B., Measelle, J. R., Armstrong, J. M., & Essex, M. J. (2005). Trajectories of classroom externalizing behavior: Contributions of child characteristics, family characteristics, and the teacher-child relationship during the school transition. *Journal of School Psychology, 43*, 39–60. https://doi.org/10.1016/j.jsp.2004.11.003

Sims, M., Guilfoyle, A., & Parry, T. S. (2006). Children's cortisol levels and quality ofchild care provision. *Child: Care, Health and Development, 32*, 453–466. https://doi.org/10.1111/j.1365-2214.2006.00632.x

Slatcher, R. B., & Robles, T. F. (2012). Brief report: Preschoolers' everyday conflict at home and diurnal cortisol patterns. *Health Psychology, 31*, 834–838. https://doi.org/10.1037/a0026774

Soliday Hong, S. L., Howes, C., Marcella, J., Zucker, E., & Huang, Y. (2015). Quality rating and improvement systems: Validation of a local implementation in LA county and children's school-readiness. *Early Childhood Research Quarterly, 30*(part B), 227–240. https://doi.org/10.1016/j.ecresq.2014.05.001

Teachstone. (2016). *QRIS and the Classroom Assessment Scoring System*. Retrieved from http://teachstone.com/classroom-assessment-scoring-system/qris/.

van Ijzendoorn, M. H., Schuengel, C., & Bakersmans-Kranenburg, M. J. (1999). Disorganized attachment in early childhood: Meta-analysis of precursors, concomitants, and sequelae. *Development and Psychopathology, 11*, 225–249. https://doi.org/10.1017/s0954579499002035

Vandell, D. L., Belsky, J., Burchinal, M., Steinberg, L., Vandergrist, N., & NICHD Early Child Care Research Network. (2010). Do effects of early child care extend to age 15 years? Results from the NICHD Study of Early Child Care and Youth Development. *Child Development, 81*, 737–756. https://doi.org/10.1111/j.1467-8624.2010.01431.x

Vermeer, H. J., Groeneveld, M. G., Larrea, I., van Ijzendoorn, M. H., Barandiaran, A., & Linting, M. (2010). Child care quality and children's cortisol in Basque Country and the Netherlands. *Journal of Applied Developmental Psychology, 31*, 339–347. https://doi.org/10.1016/j.appdev.2010.05.001

Vermeer, H. J., & van Ijzendoorn, M. H. (2006). Children's elevated cortisol levels at childcare: A review and meta-analysis. *Early Childhood Research Quarterly, 21*, 390–401. https://doi.org/10.1016/j.ecresq.2006.07.004

Walter, F., Torres, A., & Aldebot-Green, A. (2015). *Elevating quality rating and improvement system communications: How to improve outreach to and engagement with providers, parents, policymakers, and the public*. Retrieved from https://www.childtrends.org/wp-content/uploads/2015/07/2015-30aQRISCommExecSum1.pdf.

Watamura, S. E., Donzella, B., Alwin, J., & Gunnar, M. R. (2003). Morning-to-afternoon increases in cortisol concentrations for infants and toddlers at child care: Age differences and behavioral correlates. *Child Development, 74*, 1006–1020. https://doi.org/10.1111/1467-8624.00583

Watamura, S. E., Kryzer, E. M., & Robertson, S. S. (2009). Cortisol patterns at home and child care: Afternoon differences and evening recovery in children attending very high quality full-day center-based child care. *Journal of Applied Developmental Psychology, 30*, 475–485. https://doi.org/10.1016/j.appdev.2008.12.027

Weiland, C., Ulvestad, K., Sachs, J., & Yoshikawa, H. (2013). Associations between classroom quality and children's vocabulary and executive function skills in an urban public prekindergarten program. *Early Childhood Research Quarterly, 28*, 199–209. https://doi.org/10.1016/j.ecresq.2012.12.002

Wener, C. D., Linting, M., Vermeer, H. J., & van IJzeondoorn, M. H. (2016). Do intervention programs in child care promote the quality of caregiver-child Interactions? A meta-analysis of randomized controlled trials. *Prevention Science, 17*, 259–273. https://doi.org/10.1007/s11121-015-0602-7

Williford, A. P., LoCasale-Crouch, J., Whittaker, J. V., DeCoster, J., Hartz, K. A., Carter, L. M., … Hatfield, B. E. (2017). Changing teacher-child dyadic interactions to improve preschool children's externalizing behaviors. *Child Development, 88*, 1544–1553. https://doi.org/10.1111/cdev.12703

Yudron, M., Jones, S. M., & Raver, C. C. (2014). Implications of different methods for specifying classroom composition of externalizing behavior and its relationship to social-emotional outcomes. *Early Childhood Research Quarterly, 29*, 682–691. https://doi.org/10.1016/j.ecresq.2014.07.007

Zalewski, M., Lengua, L., Thompson, S., & Kiff, C. (2016). Income, cumulative risk, and longitudinal profiles of hypothalamic–pituitary–adrenal axis activity in preschool-age children. *Development and Psychopathology, 28*, 341–353. https://doi.org/10.1017/S0954579415000474

Zalewski, M., Lengua, L. J., Kiff, C. J., & Fisher, P. A. (2012). Understanding the relation of low income to HPA-Axis functioning in preschool children: Cumulative family risk and parenting as pathways to disruptions in cortisol. *Child Psychiatry & Human Development, 43*, 924–942. https://doi.org/10.1007/s10578-y012-0304-3

Zhai, F., Waldfogel, J., & Brooks-Gunn, J. (2013). Estimating the effects of Head Start on parenting and child maltreatment. *Children and Youth Services Review, 35*, 1119–1129. https://doi.org/10.1016/j.childyouth.2011.03.008

Chapter 6
Stress, Biomarkers, and Resilience in Childhood and Adolescence: Advances in the Last Few Decades

Elizabeth J. Susman

The aim of this chapter is to discuss advances in the stress biomarker cortisol in relation to theory, findings, and individual differences in reactivity of the hypothalamic pituitary adrenal (HPA) axis endocrine system and behavior and emotions as they relate to risk and resilience. The process of positive recovering from an adverse event is referred to as resilience (Fletcher & Sarkar, 2013). Chronic exposure to atypical stress hormone levels, principally cortisol, in the prenatal period, infancy, childhood, adolescence, adulthood, or aging can have an impact on health and brain development (Lupien, McEwen, Gunnar, & Heim, 2009). A relevant specific finding is that there were curvilinear relations of income and cumulative risk to stress profiles in young children. An atypical low morning cortisol level and flattened diurnal slope were reported in children with both higher and lower incomes and cumulative risks (Zalewski, Lengua, Thompson, & Kiff, 2016). The findings point to the importance of considering the range of incomes and family environments when identifying stress sensitive children. Atypical cortisol patterns do not necessarily confer resilience in young children.

For decades now scholars have been enthralled by models and theories of how endogenous and exogenous stressors affect products of the stress system and how these effects in turn may alter development. Advances in biomarker technology have made it possible to assess stress via one possible mechanism, cortisol, using saliva, blood, urine, or hair. Delayed in articulation are theories that integrate the neurobiology of stress, cortisol, and various aspects of risk and resilience. The absence of theories is evident in the relative lack of existing empirical studies that are based on sound theory integrating biomarkers of risk and resilience. In addition to the need for specific theories is the search for mechanisms whereby exogenous

E. J. Susman, Ph.D. (✉)
Department of Biobehavioral Health, The Pennsylvania State University, University Park, PA, USA
e-mail: ejs5@psu.edu

A. W. Harrist, B. C. Gardner (eds.), *Biobehavioral Markers in Risk and Resilience Research*, Emerging Issues in Family and Individual Resilience,
https://doi.org/10.1007/978-3-030-05952-1_6

events become part of the individual's DNA, brain, stress system, and subsequent health and behavior. Understanding mechanisms whereby stress and cortisol secretion affect resilience has the potential for greatly increasing our understanding of the neurobiology underlying resilience. Thus, this report will include (1) a short history of the integration of stress biomarkers in studies of health and risk and resilience. (2) Advances in theories of biomarker science are then discussed. (3) Maltreatment will be discussed as a specific instance of how early life adversity affects cortisol secretion. (4) The report concludes with implications for the future of research on cortisol and the neurobiology of stress and resilience.

6.1 History of Stress Biomarkers in Risk and Resilience Research in Children

The need for new explanations for the causal links between stress and disease has been an ongoing mystery to solve throughout history given that the elusive cures for stress-related diseases remain constant (McEwen & Stellar, 1993). The putative links between stress and psychological processes and behavior, an idea referred to as mind-body interface, have occupied a prominent place in the history of brain, body, and behavior intersection. The dual mind-body theories of the biological stress system and disease on the one hand and psychological development and health on the other hand have waxed and waned for centuries (Harrington, 2008). Decarte espoused that the mind and body were completely separate. Cartesian dualism eventually was replaced with a more holistic approach to mind and body given a growing body of scientific approaches and empirical findings integrating mind and body. Cannon (1929) and Selye (1956) provided the foundation for understanding the dynamic and ongoing links between the mind and stressors such as illnesses and disorders. A primary question was under what conditions in the external milieu does the body respond to exogenous stressors and how do these responses differ across individuals. Hans Selye (1956) proposed a nonspecific response to stress, the general adaption syndrome (GAS). GAS considers the short- and long-term, or chronic reactions to stress, and suggests that the GAS allows the individual to adapt to a host of stressors to achieve equilibrium. Almost entirely new fields connecting stress and disease then emerged in the mid and late twentieth century: behavioral medicine, health psychology, and holistic health. The new fields were fueled by evidence partially from World War II (Yehuda et al., 1990) showing the effects of war time stress on mental and physical health. For instance, it became evident post World War II that conditions of normal life and just not combat could produce physiological changes in the stress system (Lazarus, 1993). These new fields reflected a paradigm shift from mind-body dualism toward the integration of psychological states and diseases and disorders.

Biomarkers of stress, like cortisol, eventually became popular indices to show how individuals vary on levels of physiological reactions to exogenous stressors in novel and stressful circumstances. An additional aspect of the growth of cortisol studies was the question of whether cortisol levels (stress and nonstress or basal levels) varied across individuals in comparable contexts, and how levels correlated with disease or maladaptive behavior. In addition, a growing consensus was that early adversity or early life stress (ELS) affects adult health and behavior (Taylor, Way, & Seeman, 2011). Studies of stress, aggression, and antisocial behavior as an aspect of health began in the 1980s (McBurnett, Pfiffner, & Frick, 2001) but females tended not to be included in the samples given that females are putatively less aggressive than males. Much more is known about cortisol and risk than cortisol and resilience. Antisocial behavior can include physical aggression, deviant and criminal behavior, and violence in the family environment and everyday contexts. Important to note is that the links between cortisol and antisocial behaviors are considered a process as the stress system is dynamic and constantly changing therefore making it difficult to capture a stable snapshot of the true relationship between stress, aggression, cortisol, emotions, and behavior. Cortisol has much more often been considered a risk as opposed to a resilience process and antisocial behavior.

6.2 Cortisol in the Last Few Decades

The research on cortisol as a putative index of experienced stress has grown precipitously in both quantity and quality in recent history. One of the first contemporary reviews of the stress system, cortisol and development was a meta-analysis by Dickerson and Kemeny (2004). That analysis included 208 laboratory studies of acute psychological stressors and tested a theoretical model delineating conditions capable of eliciting cortisol responses. Consistent with the theoretical model, motivated performance tasks elicited cortisol responses if they were uncontrollable or characterized by social-evaluative threat (negative evaluations), even when methodological factors and other stressor characteristics were controlled (Dickerson & Kemeny, 2004). Tasks consisting of both uncontrollable and social-evaluative elements were associated with the largest cortisol and adrenocorticotropin (ACTH) hormone changes and the longest times to recovery. The findings provided evidence that, overall, like physical stressors (e.g., electric shock), psychological stressors can activate the HPA axis. This review was oriented to lab stressors and cannot be compared to stressors in a naturalistic setting such as a family environment. Nonetheless, the findings were consistent with the animal literature (Levine, 1985) on the HPA effects of uncontrollable social threat and confirmed the belief that cortisol is responsive to multiple types of stressors.

Prior to the 1980s, the early 1990s and the Dickerson and Kemeny (2004) review studies tended to be correlational based more loosely on theoretical models relating cortisol and psychological and contextual processes. To cite the late Robert Cairns, a "paste on" approach to biology was used in studies of biomarkers and behavior. For instance, cortisol was included without sufficient theoretical justification of it as an indicator of risk for antisocial behavior. In the correlational or group difference design, there was an absence of sound theoretical approaches in keeping with the scientific process that is based on a specific theory and hypotheses derived from the theory which are tested and supported or not supported. The predominant theory was that higher cortisol was a risk for aggressive behavior. With time a new theory emerged suggesting that lower cortisol levels could be indicative of a risk for antisocial problems (e.g., McBurnett et al., 2001). It is now known that lower and higher cortisol levels can be indicative of risk or resilience processes at different developmental periods and in different contexts. For instance, considerable literature suggests that childhood and family adversity is associated with a risk for heightened HPA cortisol response in childhood that might later contribute to attenuated HPA activity in adulthood (Repetti, Robles, & Reynolds, 2011). Overall cortisol levels and resilience usually were not considered.

The life span links between cortisol and adult behavior have many moderators. For instance, high or low cortisol can be a risk or resilience marker depending on the moderator of exposure to family aggression and violence. Margolin (2005) was one of the first to develop a systematic model for intergeneration transmission of a conflictual family environment and offspring cortisol, conflict, and aggression. Youth with high exposure to family violence showed lower cortisol output during a laboratory-based conflict discussion with their parents (Saxbe, Margolin, Spies Shapiro, & Bascum, 2012). These youths were also less likely to show the normative pattern of increased cortisol reactivity to a conflict situation when they rated family aggression as more conflictual. Family aggression also interacted with cortisol reactivity in predicting youth adjustment. Adolescents from more aggressive homes who were also more cortisol reactive to the discussion reported more post-traumatic stress symptoms and more antisocial behavior. In an earlier study children who experienced childhood trauma show the opposite pattern of heightened cortisol reactivity, lower cortisol reactivity, compared to controls, when they face stressors (Heim, Newport, Mletzko, Miller, & Nemeroff, 2008). These children might be considered more resilient, the ability to bounce back from trauma, to the effects of family conflict.

Overall, patterns of cortisol as risks or resilience processes may also be passed from parents and the family environment to children. Arbel, Rodriguez, and Margolin (2016) recently showed that a childhood history of family of origin aggression (FOA) can influence HPA responsiveness during conflict discussions with their current family members later in adulthood (Arbel et al., 2016). These and other studies have advanced understanding of how early family experiences may become embedded into a child's neurobiology and later dramatically influence risk and resilience processes across development. The Arbel et al. (2016) study also shows sex variance in how early adversity can affect cortisol secretion. As suggested by the hypothesized sensitization effect, wives' experiences of FOA were associated with heightened cortisol reactivity during a conflictual family discussion. Husbands did not show a similar effect. Sex differences in reactivity are reported in multiple other studies. Reviews regarding sexual variance in cortisol levels following different stressors have also been studied extensively (e.g., Robles, Slatcher, Trombello, & McGinn, 2014; Zorn et al., 2016). Sex differences tend not to be consistent across studies.

6.3 Advances in Hypothesis Testing

The new emphasis on biomarkers of stress via cortisol concentrations provides an unprecedented opportunity for the development of new theories necessary for articulating hypotheses regarding moderators, mediators, and covariates of cortisol and behavior. As suggested above, earlier studies tended to be correlational or group difference designs largely without a strong theoretical basis for including cortisol other than it was an index of stress or stress reactivity (i.e., changes in cortisol post stressor). Simultaneously studies have begun to assess the effects of specific stressors, controlling for comparable exogenous factors like family environment, to variations in cortisol changes in laboratory paradigms. The Trier Social Stress Test (TSST) and Trier Social Stress Test for Children (TSST-C) (Buske-Kirschbaum et al., 1997; Kirschbaum, Pirke, & Hellhammer, 1993) became two standardized and popular laboratory stress paradigms for evoking a physiological, cortisol response in adults and children to a social evaluative and cognitive task. Using these standardized paradigms across studies, specific hypotheses could be formulated and individuals could be compared in terms of different reactions to a standardized stimulus (See also Dickerson & Kemeny, 2004). Investigators also became sensitive to age variations in cortisol responses to stressors. To begin to test developmental hypotheses, in very young infants, Gunnar, Porter, Wolf, Rigatuso, and Larson (1995) investigated the relations among neonatal stress (a heel stick) and its link to subsequent temperament 6 months later. Greater reactivity to the heel stick (more crying, shorter heart periods (beat to beat), slower vagal tone, and higher cortisol) was associated with lower "Distress to Limitations" temperament at 6 months. The findings were consistent with the hypothesis that the capacity to react strongly to an aversive stimulus effects better neurobehavioral organization in the newborn. Specifically, recovery measures of cardiac activity (i.e., EKG and behavioral state) were correlated with baseline (newborn) measures indicating the strong self-righting characteristics of the healthy newborn. Finally, vagal tone and salivary cortisol measures were not significantly related suggesting the importance of assessing both cardiovascular sympathetic nervous system (SNS) and HPA axis stress systems in the ontogeny of stress-temperament relations. One might conclude from these earlier studies that individual differences in response to a stressor (i.e., the heel stick) in young infants may strongly influence later temperament. In addition, a strong neonatal cortisol response characterized by an increase in cortisol appeared to be a resilience factor and was conducive to later desirable temperament.

In other studies, in the early 1980s, we formulated similar hypotheses in adolescents versus infants. The question was whether strong individual variations existed in pubertal age adolescents in their reactions to a stressor, a phlebotomy procedure (Susman et al., 1987). Adolescents have been speculated to become more sensitive to stressors during the pubertal years, between ages 9 and 15, than in earlier childhood. A second question also was whether variations in cortisol response to a painful procedure predicted antisocial behavior 1 year later. In the Susman et al. (1987) study, the stressor was a phlebotomy procedure done by a nurse practitioner to obtain blood for a larger study of gonadal and adrenal hormones and behavior in young adolescents (Nottelmann et al., 1987; Susman et al., 1987). The phlebotomy procedure was carefully standardized across individuals and occasions of measurement by using the same nurse practitioner and the same experiment room. Intra- and interindividual, group differences in cortisol reactivity in the challenging situation were identified: some adolescents increased, some did not change, and others decreased in serum cortisol during the phlebotomy procedure. Adolescents in the increased cortisol reactivity group reported more behavior problems (antisocial acting out) and symptoms of depression than did adolescents who do not change or decreased in cortisol reactivity 1 year later. These intraindividual and group difference findings were some of the first to hypothesize and demonstrate cortisol reactivity under stressful conditions as a risk for later antisocial behavior. It should be noted that these findings were generated in a laboratory setting and used blood serum as opposed to saliva, casting a warning about the findings regarding ecological validity. This report suggested that enhanced cortisol reactivity be considered a risk for antisocial behavior in young adolescents but with the evolution of studies it was shown that increased reactivity, a reputed risk at one point in the life span can be a resilience factor at other periods of the life span. See below and above for examples (e.g., Shirtcliff & Essex, 2008).

As the number of studies that included cortisol increased, reviewers became increasingly demanding of the need to move beyond correlational studies and engage in research with theory-driven hypotheses. Questions regarding the validity and stability of the various measures of cortisol also become an essential element for reviewers to consider for publishing in reputable journals. The inclusion of reliable and valid indices of cortisol became more important as studies emerged with contradictory findings. The issue of inconsistency remains a problem in published studies of cortisol and more systematic methodological studies need to be done to identify the causes and scope of the inconsistency. An example of the research and development that needs to be done with cortisol biomarkers can be found in Stalder et al. (2016) and their work regarding the cortisol awakening response (CAR), an increasingly popular index of HPA functioning. In 2016, Stalder et al. (2016) reviewed the literature on the CAR using a Consensus Conference method and made specific recommendations for improving the validity and reliability of CAR. (See below.)

The questions regarding cortisol are turning now to mechanisms at the behavioral, genetic, neurotransmitter, brain, family, and HPA axis levels regarding how an exogenous event affects the neurobiological stress system and an outcome like antisocial behavior. Exposure to early adversity and trauma is a mechanism in the explanation of the findings regarding low cortisol level or low reactivity cortisol in youth currently experiencing adversity. It has been noted that individuals exposed to early adversity such as disrupted families, conflict within the family, maltreatment, sexual abuse, or psychopathology (e.g., Anda et al., 2006; Lopez-Duran, Olson, Hajal, Felt, & Vazquez, 2009) have lower cortisol levels. This phenomenon is referred to as the attenuation hypothesis (Susman, 2006) and suggests that under chronic stressful conditions, the HPA axis downregulates thereby reducing HPA activation as a mechanism for preventing stress-related diseases under chronic adverse conditions. Attenuated cortisol in maltreated youth is an illustration to support the attenuation hypothesis (Trickett, Noll, Susman, Shenk, & Putnam, 2010). This mechanism also entails sensitivity to the environment and regulation of cortisol. Some youth are more sensitive to environmental cues than others. The theoretical perspective on cortisol and sensitivity to the environment provides a comprehensive perspective on family mechanisms mediating cortisol, the environment, and timing of puberty (Ellis, Boyce, Belsky, Bakermans-Kranenburg, & van IJzendoorn, 2011). This individual difference, sensitivity perspective is noteworthy as it is highly interdisciplinary combining anthropology, pediatrics, and developmental psychology. Guided by developmental theories of biological sensitivity to context and reproductive development, Ellis and colleagues (2012) examined interactive effects of early family environments and psychobiologic reactivity to stress on the timing and tempo of puberty within the adaptive calibration model (ADM). An evolutionary based developmental theory, ADM posits that characteristics of the family environment such as high stress, father absence, and other adverse family influences lead to individual differences in the functioning of the stress response system (Del Giudice, Ellis, & Shirtcliff, 2011). The notion is that the stress response system has three primary functions: (1) coordinates the organism's allostatic response to physical and psychosocial challenges; (2) encodes and filters information about the organism's environment, mediating the organism's openness to environmental inputs; and (3) regulates the organism's physiology and behavior in a broad range of fitness-relevant areas (e.g., defensive behaviors, competitive risk-taking, attachment, affiliation, and reproductive functioning). The information encoded by the stress system during development feeds back on the long-term calibration of the system itself, resulting in adaptive individual differences in behavior (Del Guidice et al., 2011). An empirical study based on this model hypothesized that heightened biological sensitivity (higher cortisol) to the environment would predict lesser quality parental relationships (Ellis, Shirtcliff, Boyce, Deardorff, and Essex, 2011). As predicted by the ADM, children displaying heightened biological sensitivity to the family context (i.e., higher cortisol stress reactivity) and better quality parent–child relationships forecast slower initial pubertal tempo and later pubertal timing. In contrast, lower quality parent–child relationships forecast the opposite pattern, faster puberty. No such effects emerged among less context-sensitive children. Implications can be drawn from this model one of which is that parenting quality does make a difference in the highly entrained genetic processes that guide the onset and timing of puberty. The findings also suggest intervention implications. Parents in low quality family environments with sensitive children might gain from early guidance regarding adopting more positive parenting to avoid both conflict and early timing of puberty although timing of puberty may be much more difficult to change. ADM is an excellent illustration of how hypotheses regarding risk and resilience processes within the family have advanced in the last few decades.

Recent advances in theory and research also have pointed to the importance of biology–biology interactions and behavior in the complex multilevel endocrine system. Susman et al. (2017) used an interdisciplinary integration of theories to consider the interaction between cortisol reactivity and diurnal testosterone and antisocial behavior. The *stress diathesis* and *sensitivity to the environment*theories were used to consider the interaction of cortisol reactivity and diurnal testosterone. The stress diathesis theory suggests that certain individual psychological characteristics (vulnerabilities) are risks for later psychopathology. An innovation of the current study was that a hormone, cortisol, was considered a biological risk as opposed to psychological or family contextual risk for antisocial behavior. Low and high levels of cortisol reactivity were considered vulnerabilities, or risks, for antisocial behavior. The argument was that the vulnerability of cortisol reactivity will interact with the larger neurobiological context of puberty to influence antisocial behavior. The specific marker of the endocrine environment was testosterone, a key hormone of the endocrine environment of puberty. Testosterone has a long history of being associated with antisocial behavior (Archer, 2006; van Goozen, Fairchild, Snoek, & Harold, 2007) and also is one of the primary hormones responsible for changes in secondary sex characteristics and other physical changes of puberty. Cortisol and testosterone both have energizing properties that can be oriented toward aggressive or externalizing behaviors. Specifically, testosterone was considered to have energizing characteristics via the serotonergic system (Montoya, Terburg, Bos, & van Honk, 2012). Diurnal (awakening level) testosterone was considered the endocrine context as morning testosterone tends to be an accurate index of puberty and is higher in the morning even in pubertal age children. The biological context (testosterone-puberty vs. family context) was hypothesized to interact with the preexisting vulnerability of cortisol sensitivity. Thus, it was argued that cortisol reactivity is a vulnerability for antisocial behavior in interaction with the pubertal context of testosterone and will predict antisocial behavior. The hypothesis was that cortisol reactivity (vulnerability) would interact with diurnal testosterone to predict antisocial behavior across 6 and 12 months. The findings were as predicted. The interactions of cortisol reactivity and diurnal testosterone showed that in the *low* cortisol reactivity group, antisocial behavior (total antisocial behavior, attention problems, oppositional defiant disorder (ODD) symptoms, rule break and aggressive problems) was higher in the low and medium testosterone groups than in the high testosterone group. In contrast, in the *high* cortisol reactivity group, antisocial behavior (total antisocial behavior, attention problems, ODD symptoms, rule breaking and aggressive behavior) was higher in the high testosterone group than in low testosterone group primarily in boys. The implication of the findings is that parents and teachers should be cognizant of the possibility of changes in reactivity to stressors during the early, often stressful, puberty-related testosterone changes.

6.4 Trauma, Early Life Events (ELS), and Biomarkers

Major advances in the HPA/cortisol and risk and resilience literatures have to do with the role of trauma in HPA activation. Beginning with Yehuda, links were demonstrated between early life stress (ELS), trauma, and PTSD. These three seemingly similar phenomenon are all related to aberration in the HPA axis and will be considered together. ELS increases risk for both adult traumatization and post-traumatic stress disorder (PTSD). Yehuda et al. (2010) suggest that HPA axis is a pathway through which childhood trauma/ELS may increase risk for adult traumatization and post-traumatic stress disorder (PTSD). In addition to the diagnoses of PTSD, ELS is related to anxiety, depression, and health problems in adulthood (e.g., Lehrner et al., 2016). Adult PTSD may also reflect a continuation of a response to an earlier exposure to adversity. Such is the case for the links between childhood abuse and later HPA axis functioning (Trickett et al., 2010). Given similarities between neuroendocrine aspects of PTSD and ELS, such as in reduced cortisol signaling and glucocorticoid receptor (GR) responsiveness, some aspects of the biology of PTSD may reflect biological correlates of risk (Yehuda et al. 2010) in youth. An additional leap in the understanding of neurobiology of ELS and PTSD is the role of methylation. Methylation refers to an epigenetic mechanism whereby cells control the expression of genes. ELS may produce some of the PTSD-associated changes in glucocorticoid responsiveness through epigenetic mechanisms. The associated changes may contribute to enduring changes in stress responsiveness as well as enhanced risk for adult exposure to trauma and PTSD. These explanations run parallel to explaining lower cortisol levels in traumatized children and adolescents referred to in the attenuation hypothesis (Susman, 2006). Parenthetically, an early life event does not require a prolonged exposure to trauma for its effects to be long-lasting.

The effects of maltreatment as trauma and ELS are often referred to synonymously and have become important concepts in the child abuse literature. Unfortunately, the longitudinal studies needed to describe maltreatment, ELS, and HPA axis functioning are scarce. The exception is an 18-year longitudinal study of sexually abused girls across childhood and adolescence (Trickett et al., 2010). The girls were assessed on biological and psychological indices at six time points from childhood through adolescence and into adulthood. The aim was to assess whether childhood sexual abuse disrupted the developmental trajectory of HPA activity. The findings clearly showed that relative to comparison females, the linear trend (trajectory) for abused females was significantly less steep (less increase over time) when cortisol was examined from age 6 to age 30. The findings remained after controlling for theoretically relevant variables like depression, anxiety, and obesity. As a direct test of the attenuation hypothesis, supplemental analyses of time since disclosure of abuse indicated that cortisol levels were initially significantly higher and slopes were significantly less steep in sexually abused trajectory. But the trajectory changed with cortisol levels becoming lower at around puberty. This finding provided the first longitudinal evidence to support the hypothesis that maltreatment influences the psychobiology of cortisol functioning, and that there is a normative nonstress cortisol increase over time in healthy, maltreated girls.

The effects of ELS in the form of sexual abuse can have effects that are widespread, affecting not only the HPA stress axis but also the neuroendocrine reproductive, hypothalamic pituitary gonadal (HPG) axis. The HPA and HPG axes interact to affect both reproduction and stress responses. Specifically, cortisol putatively suppresses the HPG system at various points in the axes. For instance, adrenocorticotropin hormone (ACTH) and cortisol can suppress the HPA reproductive axis. Applied to the stress of maltreatment, the HPG axis should be suppressed by the onset of puberty given classical endocrine thinking about high cortisol and suppression of the reproductive system. Rather than a delay in timing of puberty perhaps secondary to high cortisol, studies of the timing of puberty in sexually abused girls showed earlier timing of puberty (Noll et al., 2017). Trickett et al. (2010) and Noll et al. (2017) were the first to show in their well-designed longitudinal studies that sexual maltreatment appears to lead to earlier activation of the reproductive axis responsible for onset and progression of puberty in girls. Noll et al. (2017) reported that a history of sexual abuse was related to earlier pubertal timing: 8 months earlier for breasts and 12 months earlier for pubic hair. This study confirms a relationship between exposure to childhood sexual abuse and earlier pubertal onset. Various explanations have been given for this earlier puberty: conflict in the family environment, father absence, obesity. Results highlight the possibility that, due to earlier onset, sexual abuse survivors may be at increased risk for psychosocial difficulties, menstrual and fertility problems, and even reproductive cancers due to prolonged, lifetime exposure to sex hormones.

The Noll et al. (2017) and Trickett et al. (2010) reports are unique in a number of ways; the study is theoretically driven, is based on a long-term longitudinal design, the sexually abused girls are carefully matched with the comparison girls and relevant covariates are included to rule out competing explanations (e.g., ethnicity, obesity, father absence/presence). Of note is that in previous studies few used standard indices of stage of puberty as defined by Tanner and colleagues. In addition, sexually abused and comparison youth (not abused) were carefully compared and the comparison group was matched with the abused group on a number of relevant dimensions.

The observed effects of sexual maltreatment on brain development can be inferred from variations in timing of puberty and attenuation of cortisol in sexually abused girls (Trickett et al., 2010). Implicated brain structures and functions include reliable morphological alterations in anterior cingulate, dorsal lateral prefrontal and orbitofrontal cortex, corpus callosum and adult hippocampus, and enhanced amygdala response to expressive faces and low striatal response to anticipated rewards (Teicher & Samson, 2016). There is also speculation that the interconnecting pathways in these effects of maltreatment have sensitive developmental periods in which they are vulnerable (See also Anda et al., 2006). These reports advance the science of ELS, the HPA axis and brain development, and show that HPA axis functioning is a mechanism involved stress reactive system.

An important consideration in studies of risk and resilience in trauma and ELS studies, including maltreatment, is the developmental age of onset of trauma and how trauma differentially affects stress and development across the life span. As individuals age their ability to cope with trauma generally increases but this assertion is in no way consistent in empirical studies. It is known that HPA axis is sensitive to stress-related trauma throughout development (Lupien et al., 2009). There is also new research showing that timing of childhood trauma is related to differences in later HPA axis functioning. Kuhlman, Vargas, Geiss, and Lopez-Duran (2015) examined the association between age of first trauma and HPA axis salivary cortisol response to a cold pressor test, the CAR and diurnal regulation at home across two consecutive weekdays in boys and girls. Timing of exposure is also related to diverging patterns of diurnal cortisol regulation for males and females with delayed recovery from peak reactivity to a cold pressor test. Later exposure resulted in fewer consequences in later development. In brief, the HPA axis appears susceptible to developing acute stress dysregulation when exposed to trauma during infancy, whereas the consequences appear to be lessened with later exposure. The findings are indicative of early sensitivity of the developing stress system.

6.5 Implications

6.5.1 Implications for Understanding Family Resilience

The findings presented above point to several theoretical and methodological issues that are relevant to future research in family resilience. Of note is that an interdisciplinary model or theory is essential for combining biomarkers and resilience in family research. When scholars attempt interdisciplinary projects, efforts often fall short because one discipline dominates or participants fail to create a common language and goals to carry out the research. An interdisciplinary perspective is especially important in research on the HPA axis and family processes as cortisol is derived from complex systems and interactions involving endocrine, autonomic, and behavioral systems (Chrousos & Gold, 1992) requiring different bodies of knowledge and different clinical expertise. Specifically, it is essential to possess a basic anatomic and physiologic understanding of the HPA axis system. If individuals are not informed of the nature of HPA axis functioning and a particular domain of family functioning, then consultants and collaborators should be garnered to avoid gross errors in technique for collecting saliva, blood, urine, or hair for cortisol (Stalder et al., 2017), sampling intervals, analysis for the saliva/blood/hair, and interpretation of the findings.

Breakout Box 6.1: Focus on Practice

Having spent many years now practicing pediatric developmental medicine, I can say without hesitation that close collaboration between myself and other specialized health care providers has been a vital part of my practice. Assessing children with severe developmental delays that are often times due to chromosomal abnormalities, anoxic brain injuries, or have no clearly identifiable etiology can be a frustrating venture, even more so in the presence of complicating comorbidities such as seizure activity, feeding issues, and social components that have previously limited care. One particular case comes to mind regarding a young girl who had been severely neglected in her infancy. When she first presented to my clinic with newly assigned foster parents at 2½ years of age, she was underweight, spoke no intelligible words and could only ambulate with great difficulty. What was clearly apparent early on was that this child had significant motor and speech delays. On review of her limited birth records there was a history of maternal drug abuse, limited prenatal care, and an anoxic brain injury sustained during delivery. She was lost to follow-up after only three visits to a primary care practitioner. Needless to say, there were multiple clinical aspects that would need to be addressed. I wish I could say that hers is a unique story, but such is not the case. But cases such as this illustrate the need for a multi-faceted, interdisciplinary approach. With the help of speech therapy professionals, occupational therapists, social workers, a neurologist, my own assessments, and an attentive primary care provider to coordinate care between a growing list of providers, a cohesive team with a unified goal was created. Though the term was initially coined to refer to child rearing, to say that "it takes a village" is an appropriate way to characterize the type of care needed for complex patients in many different medical settings. The importance of fostering an atmosphere, which encourages and supports the process of an interdisciplinary treatment plan, cannot be overstated.

Note: This was written from the combined sentiments of multiple healthcare providers to include pediatricians, speech therapy, a developmental pediatrician, and occupational/physical therapy.

6.5.2 Implications for Research Policy on Biomarkers and Family Resilience

An in-depth review that considers all the relevant issues with regard to including cortisol and resilience in families is well beyond the scope of this report. Nonetheless a number of considerations are important to mention. Of primary importance is that the research hypothesis will guide the relevant theory and method of assessment of cortisol. Cortisol can be measured in saliva, blood, urine, and hair, and each method requires unique expertise in regard to sampling, storage, and analysis. Arising from the medical model, traditionally blood (usually serum) was the preferred substance for assaying for cortisol concentrations for diagnostic purposes. A major problem with using blood for cortisol in family studies is the invasive nature of obtaining blood via phlebotomy or blood sticks and the changes in cortisol related to the stress of having blood drawn. Then came the discovery that the stress hormone, cortisol, could also be assayed in saliva with validity and reliability. In 1994, Kirschbaum and Hellhammer (1994) declared that saliva cortisol was a valid and reliable reflection of the respective unbound hormone in blood. Hence, saliva cortisol like serum became prominent in applied research related to emotional distress or cognitive challenges as opposed to diagnostic assessments. For the last 25 years Granger and colleagues, first at Penn State and now at University of California, Irvine, have been confirming the validity and reliability of cortisol salivary assays and doing the research and development on more accurate ways of collecting and analyzing saliva for assays (https://www.salimetrics.com). This careful research and development work led to even more advances in cortisol research with families as saliva became more acceptable to participants and in published studies. With advances in cortisol measurement, an even more important consideration was what theories underlie the collection of saliva; the theory dictates the determinant of the actual biological substance and sampling method that should be used to test the hypotheses. For instance, if the theory suggests that one wants to assess cortisol diurnal variations in the HPA axis then the CAR (Stalder et al., 2016), samples would be the measure of choice given its association with psychiatric disorders characterized by high cortisol levels in the morning as in the case of depression. If the interest is in change in cortisol level following a stressor, then measuring cortisol prior to and after a known stressor, like the TSST, is the measure of choice. In addition, theories of chronic stress necessitate different measures like chronic stress and hair given that hair samples require a longer time frame for the accumulation of cortisol in hair fibers (Stalder & Kirschbaum, 2012; Ullmann, Barthlet, Petrowski, Stalder, & Bornstein, 2016). Hair samples provide a retrospective reflection of integrated cortisol secretion over periods of several months. Given its newness as a cortisol biomarker there is less information on its validity and reliability. Helpful is a recent review of the evidence on hair samples as an index of cortisol. With the accumulation of studies supportive evidence is growing suggesting the validity of hair cortisol as an index of long-term systemic cortisol levels and its reliability across repeated measurements and its robustness to a range of potential confounding influences. Given that family conflict may take place over an extended period of time, hair samples for cortisol seem highly relevant.

Developmental differences in cortisol across the life span are equally important considerations in research on resilience. Cortisol is known to vary across the life span with increases in cortisol at birth, a decrease thereafter and a less dramatic increase during puberty (Susman et al, 2017). Different considerations must be applied in studies that include pregnant women. Cortisol rises from the early weeks of pregnancy until delivery but most of the cortisol during pregnancy is bound to corticotropin binding globulin (CBG) making it impossible to compare values during pregnancy to values in nonpregnant states. If cortisol is collected during pregnancy, it is prudent to also assay for CBG making it possible to calculate the bound and unbound portion of cortisol during pregnancy. Failure to consider developmental differences or other conditions like pregnancy can result in serious interpretative problems, thus invalidating the findings for future interventions.

6.6 Conclusions and Future Directions

The future of cortisol biomarkers is likely to consist of advances in improving the validity of cortisol assays and study designs for answering relevant questions regarding family resilience. A major concern regarding cortisol measures is the inconsistency in findings in studies on cortisol and emotions, behaviors (antisocial behavior), and family functioning. For instance, low levels of cortisol and higher levels of aggressive behavior are expected but are not always the case. The inconsistency may arise partially because current research designs are not well equipped to capture the dynamic changes in cortisol across minutes, the 24-h circadian rhythms, days and seasons. Dynamic changes also occur in family functioning and resilience may vary with these dynamic characteristics.

Inconsistencies also arise from similar studies because of the following: saliva is collected in stress and nonstress contexts, mean levels are used over a shorter or longer period of assessment, across the diurnal cycle. Additionally, cortisol is collected at different times across the 24-h circadian cycle. These potential problems are recognized but rarely explored in detail to root out the source of variability until recently. Under the auspices of the Psychoneuroendocrine Society, a consensus group of scholars was assembled and a review of the cortisol awakening response (CAR) was conducted (Stalder et al., 2016). This review and critique provides a state-of-the-art framework for improving the reliability and validity of the morning awakening response (CAR). A CAR has ecological validity as saliva is collected in the home, but it lacks direct scientific scrutiny which can be problematic as the validity of CAR measurement relies on the compliant participant. Saliva for CAR must be collected at exact times beginning at the moment of awakening. Even in compliant participants the prescribed time of collecting a CAR cortisol can be off time. If the first sample is delayed more than 15 min after awakening then the levels yield a false, first morning sample as well as a falsely low CAR. To resolve this problem, Stalder et al. (2016) suggest objective indices of the timing of the sample. These include a daily log, polysonography, or a less expensive alternative wrist actigraphy. An important theoretical issue for future research and an implication of the review is that the CAR is considered a distinct aspect of the HPA circadian rhythm. It does not necessarily correlate with cortisol levels at other times of the day (Bouma, Riese, Ormel, Verhulst, & Oldehinkel, 2009). Specifically, it does not relate to cortisol reactivity levels in response to laboratory induced stressors (Bouma et al., 2009). Interestingly, in an early study, the CAR was found to be closely related to the cortisol rise following ACTH-challenge suggesting that its secretion may be influenced by the maximal capacity of the adrenal cortex to produce cortisol (Schmidt-Reinwald et al., 1999). Therefore, the CAR is a useful index to use when one is interested in the maximal response of the HPA axis such as in psychiatric disorders like depression. Failure to comply with the guidelines may obstruct tests of specific hypotheses based on theories of HPA axis functions and behavior related to family resilience. Importantly, consensus reports on other methods used to assess diurnal variations in cortisol could improve the science of stress and resilience to a large degree. A review and consensus report of diurnal variations and cortisol levels like that of Stalder et al. (2016) for the CAR will improve decisions as to whether one should intervene to change cortisol levels and perhaps improve resilience.

This chapter reviewed a limited set of studies to demonstrate advances in the science of the biomarker cortisol. It is encouraging to report that cortisol measures now are considered in families as well as in individuals. Family scientists have long been interested in the effects of family relationships on subsequent psychological and physical health (Repetti et al., 2011). Negative social experiences, especially in family contexts, contribute to the dysregulation of set-points and thresholds of biological stress reactivity that can affect long-term adaptation and adjustment.

Current research shows the theoretical pathways whereby interventions may reduce mental and physical health risks and improve resilience in families. Ha and Granger (2016) pictorially represent a model for intervention that may be used to prevent risk or enhance resilience. The model indicates that family stress and conflict can lead to HPA and sympathetic nervous system (SNS) activity in the child, HPA activity in the parent and child adjustment. Finally, improved family relationships can influence electrophysiological activity, better attunement/co-regulation, and HPA and SNS activity. Ha and Granger (2016) suggest that intervention in the form of supportive relationships leads to improved family relationships and better adjustment. Other family studies show convincingly that neurotransmitters can be altered by family intervention. Specifically, Brody et al. (2009) showed that the serotonin transporter 5-HTTLPR status (presence of 1 or 2 copies of the s allele) was linked with increases in youth substance use over time. The association was greatly reduced when youths received high levels of involved-supportive parenting. If the Brody model continues to receive empirical support, then it may have widespread applicability in future biomarker research for reducing stress-related risk and increasing resilience in families. Importantly, Brody's research shows that even genetic-based processes are modifiable and can be changed through experimental interventions. It follows then that family-based, resilience interventions may change characteristics of HPA functioning and therefore enhance resilience.

The models and theories for the assessment, analysis, and conclusions regarding the biomarker cortisol and risk and resilience have implications for research, advocacy, and practice. First, for centuries it was assumed that anything biological was genetic and not modifiable. Now it is known that genetics as well as hormones are modifiable through intervention at the individual and family levels (Brody et al., 2016). Second, advocates for enhancing family resilience might profit from a more comprehensive holistic approach to understand stress, health, and behavior by including cortisol and other biomarkers. Scientists now have a sound theoretical basis for including not just cortisol in studies of resilience but a range of biological biomarkers of genetics, endocrinology, immunology, and brain development. Third, in practice therapists can not only use methods (e.g., mindfulness) to change the stress system and family functioning but genetic influences may also be changed through epigenetics which in turn may change resilience in future generations. Studies of stress and biomarkers are highly important to family scientists given the relevance of biomarker aberrations for family functioning. Education and public service information should be discriminated that will encourage therapists, families, and individuals to consider biomarkers in future efforts to reduce family risk and increase family resilience.

Questions for Thought and Discussion

1. What is the difference between a theory and a model? Describe the history of theories in the biomarker cortisol.
2. You are giving a lecture to a group of parents on adolescents and stress. Describe how one might measure stress from physiological perspective.
3. What is a biomarker and what is most prominent biomarker used in research on stress? How is it measured and why?
4. Elaborate on some theories/notions about how the biomarker cortisol might profitably be used in understanding stress and resilience.
5. What is an interdisciplinary perspective and why is it important in understanding biology and resilience?

Glossary

Adaptive Calibration Model (ADM) An evolutionary based developmental theory that posits that characteristics of the family environment such as high stress and adverse family influences lead to individual differences in the functioning of the stress response system.

Child Maltreatment Physical, sexual, or psychological mistreatment or neglect of a child or children, especially by a parent or other caregiver.

Cortisol A steroid hormone, in the glucocorticoid class of hormones. When used as a medication, it is known as hydrocortisone.

Cortisol Awakening Response (CAR) An increase of about 50% in cortisol levels occurring 20–30 min *after* awakening in the morning in some people.

Diurnal variations Fluctuations that occur every day.

Hypothalamic Pituitary Adrenal Axis A complex set of direct influences and feedback interactions among three endocrine glands: the hypothalamus, the pituitary gland (a pea-shaped structure located below the thalamus), and the adrenal glands (small, cone shaped organs on top of the kidneys).

Hypothalamic Pituitary Gonadal (HPG) Axis The HPG axis refers to the hypothalamus, pituitary gland, and gonadal glands. These glands often act in concert to play a critical part in the development and regulation of the reproductive and immune systems.

Methylation Methylation refers to an epigenetic mechanism whereby cells control the expression of genes.

Post-Traumatic Stress Syndrome/Disorder (PTSS/PTSD) Refers an emotional problem that can develop after a person is exposed to a traumatic event, such as sexual assault, warfare, traffic collisions, or other threats on a person's life.

References

Anda, R. F., Felitti, V. J., Bremner, J. D., Walker, J. D., Whitfield, C. H., Perry, B. D., ... Giles, W. H. (2006). The enduring effects of abuse and related adverse experiences in childhood. *European Archives of Psychiatry and Clinical Neuroscience, 256*, 174–186. https://doi.org/10.1007/s00406-005-0624-4

Arbel, R., Rodriguez, A. J., & Margolin, G. (2016). Cortisol reactions during family conflict discussions: Influences of wives' and husbands' exposure to family-of-origin aggression. *Psychology of Violence, 6*, 519–528. https://doi.org/10.1037/a003971

Archer, J. (2006). Testosterone and human aggression: An evaluation of the challenge hypothesis. *Neuroscience & Biobehavioral Reviews, 30*, 319–345. https://doi.org/10.1016/j.neubiorev.2004.12.007

Bouma, E. M., Riese, H., Ormel, J., Verhulst, F. C., & Oldehinkel, A. J. (2009). Adolescents' cortisol responses to awakening and social stress; effects of gender, menstrual phase and oral contraceptives. The TRAILS study. *Psychoneuroendocrinology, 34*, 884–893. https://doi.org/10.1016/j.psyneuen.2009.01.003

Brody, G. H., Beach, S. R., Philibert, R. A., Chen, Y. F., Lei, M. K., Murry, V. M., & Brown, A. C. (2009). Parenting moderates a genetic vulnerability factor in longitudinal increases in youths' substance use. *Journal of Consulting and Clinical Psychology, 77*, 1–11. https://doi.org/10.1111/j.1467-8624.2009.01288.x

Brody, G. H., Yu, T., Miller, G. E., et al. (2016). Resilience in Adolescence, Health, and Psychosocial Outcomes. *Pediatrics, 138*, e20161042

Buske-Kirschbaum, A., Jobst, S., Wustmans, A., Kirschbaum, C., Rauh, W., & Hellhammer, D. (1997). Attenuated free cortisol response to psychosocial stress in children with atopic dermatitis. *Psychosomatic Medicine, 59*, 419–426. https://doi.org/10.1097/00006842-199707000-00012

Cannon, W. B. (1929). *Bodily changes in pain, hunger, fear and rage*. New York, NY: Appleton.

Chrousos, G. P., & Gold, P. W. (1992). The concepts of stress and stress system disorders: Overview of physical and behavioral homeostasis. *The Journal of the American Medical Association, 267*, 1244–1252. https://doi.org/10.1001/jama.1992.03480090092034

Del Giudice, M., Ellis, B. J., & Shirtcliff, E. A. (2011). The adaptive calibration model of stress responsivity. *Neuroscience & Biobehavioral Reviews, 35*, 1562–1592. https://doi.org/10.1016/j.neubiorev.2010.11.007

Dickerson, S. S., & Kemeny, M. E. (2004). Acute stressors and cortisol responses: A theoretical integration and synthesis of laboratory research. *Psychological Bulletin, 130*, 355–391. https://doi.org/10.1037/0033-2909.130.3.355

Ellis, B. J., Boyce, W. T., Belsky, J., Bakermans-Kranenburg, M. J., & van IJzendoorn, M. H. (2011). Differential susceptibility to the environment: An evolutionary–neurodevelopmental theory. *Development and Psychopathology, 23*, 7–28. https://doi.org/10.1017/S0954579410000611

Ellis, B. J., Shirtcliff, E. A., Boyce, T., Deardorff, D., & Essex, M. J. (2011). Quality of early family relationships and timing and tempo of puberty. *Development and Psychopathology, 23*, 85–91. https://doi.org/10.1017/S095457941000066

Ellis, B. J., Del Giudice, M., Dishion, T. J., Figueredo, A. J., Gray, P., Griskevicius, V., ... & Wilson, D. S. (2012). The evolutionary basis of risky adolescent behavior: Implications for science, policy, and practice. *Developmental Psychology, 48*, 598–623. https://doi.org/10.1037/a0026220

Fletcher, D., & Sarkar, M. (2013). Psychological resilience: A review and critique of definitions, concepts, and theory. *European Psychologist, 18*, 12–23. https://doi.org/10.1027/1016-9040/a000124

Gunnar, M. R., Porter, F. L., Wolf, C. M., Rigatuso, J., & Larson, M. C. (1995). Neonatal stress reactivity: Predictions to later emotional temperament. *Child Development, 66*, 1–13. https://doi.org/10.2307/1131186

Ha, T., & Granger, D. A. (2016). Family relations, stress, and vulnerability: Biobehavioral implications for prevention and practice. *Developmental Psychobiology, 65*, 9–23. https://doi.org/10.1016/j.yhbeh.2016.11.018

Harrington, A. (2008). *The cure within: A history of mind-body medicine*. New York, NY: Norton.

Heim, C., Newport, D. J., Mletzko, T., Miller, A. H., & Nemeroff, C. B. (2008). The link between childhood trauma and depression: Insights from HPA axis studies in humans. *Psychoneuroendocrinology, 33*, 693–710. https://doi.org/10.1016/j.psyneuen.2008.03.008

Kirschbaum, C., & Hellhammer, D. H. (1994). Salivary Cortisol in Psychoneuroendocrine Research. *Psychoneuroendocrinology, 19*, 313–333. http://dx.doi.org/10.1016/0306-4530(94)90013-2

Kirschbaum, C., Pirke, K. M., & Hellhammer, D. H. (1993). The 'Trier Social Stress Test'—A tool for investigating psychobiological stress responses in a laboratory setting. *Neuropsychobiology, 28*, 76–81. https://doi.org/10.1159/000119004

Kuhlman, K. R., Vargas, I., Geiss, E. G., & Lopez-Duran, N. L. (2015). Age of trauma onset and HPA axis dysregulation among trauma-exposed youth. *Journal of Traumatic Stress, 28*, 572–579. https://doi.org/10.1016/j.psyneuen.2015.10.010

Lazarus, R. S. (1993). From psychological stress to the emotions: A history of changing outlooks. *Annual Review of Psychology, 44*, 1–21. https://doi.org/10.1146/annurev.ps.44.020193.000245

Lehrner, A., Flory, J. D., Bierer, L. M., Makotkine, I., Marmar, C. R., & Yehuda, R. (2016). Sexual dysfunction and neuroendocrine correlates of posttraumatic stress disorder in combat veterans: Preliminary findings. *Psychoneuroendocrinology, 63*, 271–275. https://doi.org/10.1016/j.psyneuen.2015.10.015

Levine, S. (1985). A definition of stress? In G. P. Moburg (Ed.), *Animal stress* (pp. 51–69). New York, NY: Springer. https://doi.org/10.1007/978-1-4614-7544-6_4

Lopez-Duran, N. L., Olson, S. L., Hajal, N. J., Felt, B. T., & Vazquez, D. M. (2009). Hypothalamic pituitary adrenal axis functioning in reactive and proactive aggression in children. *Journal of Abnormal Child Psychology, 37*, 169–182. https://doi.org/10.1007/s10802-008-9263-3

Lupien, S. J., McEwen, B. S., Gunnar, M. R., & Heim, C. (2009). Effects of stress throughout the lifespan on the brain, behavior and cognition. *Nature Reviews Neuroscience, 10*, 434–445. https://doi.org/10.1038/nrn2639

Margolin, G. (2005). Children's exposure to violence: Exploring developmental pathways to diverse outcomes. *Journal of Interpersonal Violence, 20*, 72–81. https://doi.org/10.1177/0886260504268371

McBurnett, K., Pfiffner, L. J., & Frick, P. J. (2001). Symptom properties as a function of ADHD type: An argument for continued study of sluggish cognitive tempo. *Journal of Abnormal Child Psychology, 29*, 207–213. https://doi.org/10.1023/A:1010377530749

McEwen, B. S., & Stellar, E. (1993). Stress and the individual: Mechanisms leading to disease. *Archives of Internal Medicine, 153*, 2093–2101. https://doi.org/10.1001/archinte.1993.00410180039004

Montoya, E. R., Terburg, D., Bos, P. A., & van Honk, J. (2012). Testosterone, cortisol, and serotonin as key regulators of social aggression: A review and theoretical perspective. *Motivation and Emotion, 36*, 65–73. https://doi.org/10.1007/s11031-011-9264-3

Noll, J., Trickett, P. K., Long, J. D., Negriff, S., Susman, E. J., Shalev, I., … Putnam, F. W. (2017). Childhood sexual abuse and early timing of puberty. *Journal of Adolescent Health, 60*, 65–71. https://doi.org/10.1016/j.adhealth.2016.09.008

Nottelmann, E. D., Susman, E. J., Inoff-Germain, G. E., Cutler, G. B., Loriaux, D. L., & Chrousos, G. P. (1987). Developmental processes in American early adolescence: Relations between adolescent adjustment problems and chronologic age, pubertal stage and puberty-related serum hormone levels. *Journal of Pediatrics, 110*, 473–480. https://doi.org/10.1016/0197-0070(87)90428-1

Repetti, R. L., Robles, T. F., & Reynolds, B. (2011). Allostatic processes in the family. *Development and Psychopathology, 23*, 921–938. https://doi.org/10.1017/S095457941100040X

Robles, T. F., Slatcher, R. B., Trombello, J. M., & McGinn, M. M. (2014). Marital quality and health: A meta-analytic review. *Psychological Bulletin, 140*, 140–187. https://doi.org/10.1037/a0031859

Saxbe, D. E., Margolin, G., Spies Shapiro, L. A., & Bascum, B. R. (2012). Does dampened physiological reactivity protect youth in aggressive family environments? *Child Development, 83, 821–830*. https://doi.org/10.1111/j.1467-8624.2012.01752.x

Schmidt-Reinwald, A., Pruessner, J. C., Hellhammer, D. H., Federenko, I., Rohleder, N., Schürmeyer, T. H., & Kirschbaum, C. (1999). The cortisol response to awakening in relation to different challenge tests and a 12-hour cortisol rhythm. *Life Sciences, 64*, 1653–1660. https://doi.org/10.1016/S0024-3205(99)00103-4

Selye, H. (1956). *The stress of life*. New York, NY: McGraw-Hill.

Shirtcliff, E., & Essex, M. (2008). Concurrent and longitudinal associations of basal and diurnal cortisol with mental health symptoms in early adolescence. *Developmental Psychobiology, 50*, 690–703. https://doi.org/10.1002/dev.20336

Stalder, T., & Kirschbaum, C. (2012). Analysis of cortisol in hair–state of the art and future directions. *Brain, Behavior, and Immunity, 26*, 1019–1029. https://doi.org/10.1016/j.bbi.2012.02.002

Stalder, T., Kirschbaum, C., Kudielka, B. M., Adam, E. K., Pruessner, J. C., Wüst, S., … Miller, R. (2016). Assessment of the cortisol awakening response: Expert consensus guidelines. *Psychoneuroendocrinology, 63*, 414–432. https://doi.org/10.1016/j.psyneuen.2015.10.010

Stalder, T., Steudte-Schmiedgen, S., Alexander, N., Klucken, T., Vater, A., Wichmann, S., … Miller, R. (2017). Stress-related and basic determinants of hair cortisol in humans: A meta-analysis. *Psychoneuroendocrinology, 77*, 261–274. https://doi.org/10.1016/j.psyneuen.2016.12.017

Susman, E. J. (2006). Psychobiology of persistent antisocial behavior: Stress, early vulnerabilities and the attenuation hypothesis. *Neuroscience and Biobehavioral Reviews, 30*, 376–389. https://doi.org/10.1016/j.neubiorev.2005.08.002

Susman, E. J., Inoff-Germain, G., Nottelmann, E. D., Loriaux, D. L., Cutler, G. B., & Chrousos, G. P. (1987). Hormones, emotional dispositions, and aggressive attributes in young adolescents. *Child Development, 58*, 1114–1134. https://doi.org/10.2307/1130551

Taylor, S. E., Way, B. M., & Seeman, T. E. (2011). Early adversity and adult health outcomes. *Development and Psychopathology, 23*, 939–954. https://doi.org/10.1017/S0954579411000411

Trickett, P. K., Noll, J. G., Susman, E. J., Shenk, C. E., & Putnam, F. W. (2010). Attenuation of cortisol across development for victims of sexual abuse. *Development and Psychopathology, 22*, 165–175. https://doi.org/10.1017/S0954579409990332

Teicher, M.H., & Samson, J.A. (2016). Annual Research Review: Enduring neurobiological effects of childhood abuse and neglect. *Journal of Child Psychology and Psychiatry, 57*, 241–66. https://doi.org/10.1111/jcpp.12507.

Ullmann, E., Barthlet, A., Petrowski, K., Stalder, T., Kirschbaum, C., & Bornstein, S. R. (2016). Pilot study of adrenal steroid hormones in hair as an indicator of chronic mental and physical stress. *Scientific Reports, 2*, 1–7. https://doi.org/10.1038/srep25842

van Goozen, S. H. M., Fairchild, G., Snoek, H., & Harold, G. T. (2007). The evidence for a neurobiological model of childhood antisocial behavior. *Psychological Bulletin, 133*, 149–182. https://doi.org/10.1037/0033-2909.133.1.149

Yehuda, R., Southwick, S. M., Nussbaum, G., Wahby, V., Giller, E. L., & Mason, J. W. (1990). Low urinary cortisol excretion in patients with posttraumatic stress disorder. *Journal of Nervous and Mental Disorders, 178*, 366–369. https://doi.org/10.1007/s00213-010-1969-6

Yehuda R, Joëls, M., Morris, R.G. (2010).The memory paradox.

Zalewski, M., Lengua, L. J., Thompson, S. F., & Kiff, C. J. (2016). Income, cumulative risk, and longitudinal profiles of hypothalamic-pituitary-adrenal axis activity in preschool-age children. *Development and Psychopathology, 28*, 341–353. https://doi.org/10.1017/S0954579415000474

Zorn, J. V., Schür, R. R., Boks, M. P., Kahn, R. S., Joëls, M., & Vinkers, C. H. (2016). Cortisol stress reactivity across psychiatric disorders: A systematic review and meta-analysis. *Psychoneuroendocrinology, 77*, 25–36. https://doi.org/10.1016/j.psyneuen.2016.11.036

Chapter 7
Challenges and Strategies for Integrating Molecular Genetics into Behavioral Science

Amanda M. Griffin, Gabriel L. Schlomer, David J. Vandenbergh, and H. Harrington Cleveland

The main body of risk and resilience research examines the influence of risk and protective factors on resilience outcomes. Risk and protective factors considered include but are not limited to child characteristics (e.g., intellectual ability, personality, and self-regulation) and environmental influences (e.g., family, interpersonal relationships, and neighborhood; Masten et al., 1999; Masten & Obradović, 2006). Risk and resilience research has been extended to include the interactions between biological risk and protective factors and environmental experiences on normative development (Cicchetti, 2010; Egeland, Carlson, & Sroufe, 1993; Luthar, Cicchetti, & Becker, 2000; Masten, 2001; Rutter, 1987, 1993, 2012). By considering biological factors, risk and resilience investigations can reevaluate resilience questions with biological influences in mind. For example, researchers can now ask: are there biological reasons why some individuals are more negatively affected by adversity than others? are there biological reasons why some individuals in adverse contexts

A. M. Griffin
University of Oregon, Eugene, OR, USA
e-mail: agriff1@uoregon.edu

G. L. Schlomer
University at Albany, State University of New York, Albany, NY, USA
e-mail: gschlomer@albany.edu

D. J. Vandenbergh
Department of Biobehavioral Health, The Pennsylvania State University, University Park, PA, USA

Institute of the Neurosciences, The Pennsylvania State University, University Park, PA, USA
e-mail: djv4@psu.edu

H. H. Cleveland (✉)
Department of Human Development and Family Science, The Pennsylvania State University, University Park, PA, USA
e-mail: hhc10@psu.edu

A. W. Harrist, B. C. Gardner (eds.), *Biobehavioral Markers in Risk and Resilience Research*, Emerging Issues in Family and Individual Resilience,
https://doi.org/10.1007/978-3-030-05952-1_7

are more impacted by the relatively few positive experiences available within these contexts? and what biological factors enable individuals to overcome adversity?

Genetic influences are one biological factor that can condition the impact of adverse contexts. Decades of research using twin and adoption designs have demonstrated substantial genetic influences on behavior (see Turkheimer, 2000), as well as the genetic moderation of environmental influences (e.g., Cleveland, 2003; Cleveland & Wiebe, 2003). In the last two decades, however, significant scientific and technological advances in genotyping have opened up new opportunities for behavioral scientists to consider genetically oriented research questions using genotyped DNA (Deoxyribonucleic acid) rather than relying on the inference of heritable effects based on twin and adoption designs (Perkel, 2008). This research has focused on examining gene-phenotype associations, where phenotypes are any measurable characteristic or trait. The pace of this work is rapidly accelerating. A recent database search found over 18,000 human molecular genetic papers published since 1960, and more than half were published within the last 10 years (Ayorech et al., 2016).

Although molecular genetic analyses are not as statistically powerful as twin and adoption designs, which can demonstrate evidence of heritable influences with relatively moderate sample sizes, adding genotypic variables to conventional datasets offers behavioral scientists opportunities that twin designs do not provide. The first advantage is straightforward. Molecular genetic research tests for associations between specific genes and phenotypes, which is potentially informative for understanding the etiology outcomes of interest. In addition, because genotypic variables can be added to any conventional dataset, this approach allows researchers to consider genetic effects on processes across the full range of independent variables, outcomes, and contextual experiences explored by behavioral science. In contrast, twin designs are inherently limited by the distribution of twins who experience contextual experiences of interest. For example, an intervention study will not have enough twins to consider genetic moderation of the intervention. Most behavioral scientists have not used twin designs due to a combination of practical limitations and the fact that behavioral scientists are interested in specific combinations of independent variables, contextual experiences, and outcomes. As a result, most behavioral scientists have, and thus most of behavioral science has, conceptualized transactions between environments and psychosocial and developmental outcomes as being solely due to environmental processes.

Projects made possible by advances in next-generation genotyping technology include collaborative international research consortia, such as the Human Genome Project (1990–2003), the HapMap Project (2002–2009), and the 1000 Genomes Project (2008–2015).[1] These projects provide publicly available catalogs of human DNA polymorphic sites, or markers (e.g., dbSNP[2]), to guide scientists conducting original genetic research as well as genotype data repositories for secondary genetic analyses (e.g., dbGaP[3]). The large-scale genotyping used in these projects was made possible by DNA microarray chips (i.e., a solid surface with microscopic DNA

[1] https://www.ncbi.nlm.nih.gov/variation/tools/1000genomes/.

[2] https://www.ncbi.nlm.nih.gov/SNP/.

[3] https://www.ncbi.nlm.nih.gov/gap.

spots) that can simultaneously genotype multiple regions of the genome. Technological advances that increased the number of genetic markers [e.g., Single Nucleotide Polymorphisms (SNPs)] on a single chip also reduced costs of genotyping. For instance, the number of SNPs that microarrays are able to assay increased from 10,000 to greater than 500,000 SNPs per chip, resulting in a 50× decrease in genotyping costs on a per-SNP basis. The continued decrease in genotyping costs has increased opportunities for behavioral scientists to integrate measured genes into their research.

GxE research is conducted through moderation analyses that examine whether the relationship between two variables differs as a function of a third variable, known as a moderator variable. This process can be conceptualized in two ways: (1) how the effect of genes on developmental outcomes is modified by environments and (2) how the effect of environments on developmental outcomes is modified by genes. Whether a gene or environment should be conceptualized as the moderator in a GxE depends on the nature of the gene, the environmental context, their association with the outcome of interest, as well as the anticipated co-action of the gene and environment on the outcomes.

Research on genetic variants offers a unique opportunity to examine individual differences in environmental reactivity with an individual characteristic that does not itself change in response to environmental experiences. In contrast, biological markers, such as folate or cortisol levels that change in response to environmental factors, allow researchers to examine the mechanisms by which adverse experiences can "get under the skin" on a physiological level. Thus, the genetic sequence provides an inferential advantage over other biological markers because between-person differences in sequence cannot be caused by environmental factors, including those operationalized within the analyses by measured variables or those that are not in the model (i.e., third variable confounds). It should be noted, however, that environmental exposures could affect epigenetic status, such as gene methylation, which alters the transcription of a gene (e.g., alter gene expression or "turning genes on or off"). Importantly, epigenetic processes play this role without changing the sequence of the DNA.

Although research using DNA has become more accessible to behavioral scientists over the last 20 years, GxE research is more complex than simply adding a DNA data collection to a conventional behavioral science study. In practice, this research endeavor requires a basic understanding of genetic markers, genetic data quality control checks, and the application of methodological strategies to increase the quality of the GxE inferences (Bakermans-Kranenburg & van Ijzendoorn, 2015; Dick et al., 2015; Salvatore & Dick, 2015; Schlomer, Cleveland, Vandenbergh, Fosco, & Feinberg, 2015; Uher & McGuffin, 2008). To assist behavioral scientists in conducting meaningful GxE research, our goal here is to present challenges associated with conducting high quality GxE research and provide strategies for addressing these challenges. Topics addressed include an abridged summary of basic aspects of molecular genetics, an overview of genetic data quality controls checks, a short review of the history of single candidate gene-by-environment (cGxE) research and the criticisms directed toward it, a framework for evaluating the quality of individual GxE studies, and a discussion of advancing GxE research through polygenic methods that aggregate the effects of multiple genetic variants. It should be noted that although gene-by-environment interaction (GxE) research can include studies that use twin and adoption designs, the primary topic of this chapter is GxE based on molecular genetics research. The notation cGxE, for which the "c" stands for candidate, can be used for this research. However, unless otherwise noted, we use the term GxE to refer to GxE research that examines molecular genetics and measured environmental variables.

7.1 Putting the G in GxE

DNA is made of a pair of nucleotide strands with bases (i.e., adenine, guanine, thymine, and cytosine) encoding the information that is transcribed into a sequence of ribonucleic acid (RNA) that is then translated to produce a protein. Although this simplified definition does not fully capture the complexities of DNA function, this DNA-to-RNA-to-protein process lies at the core of how DNA sequences influence phenotypes and is appropriately known as the Central Dogma of Molecular Biology (Crick, 1958). There are two copies, or pairs, of each double-stranded DNA molecule, called chromosomes; one copy is inherited from the mother and one from the father. Modern molecular biology techniques have shown that the two chromosomes can vary when examined at a molecular level. Alleles refer to any variation at a specific site on a pair of chromosomes, and a pair of alleles (one on each chromosome) constitutes a genotype. When collecting genotypic data, specific genetic markers (also called genetic variants) are selected in advance, usually based on one of two reasons: (1) the genetic marker has a known functional role (i.e., affects protein production) and thus might be causally related to a phenotype, or (2) the genetic marker has no known function but serves as a way to tag a chromosomal region of interest that is theorized to be related to a phenotype. Genetic markers that tag a region permit a researcher to assess variability in a larger portion of the genome by genotyping only one or a few markers in that region.

Genetic markers or variants refer to between-person differences in DNA genotype known as polymorphisms. There are different types of polymorphisms. A polymorphism can be a difference in a single nucleotide base pair (a SNP), an insertion and/or deletion of one or more base pairs (In/Del), the presence of short tandem repeats (STRs; 2–10 base pairs), or variable number of tandem repeats (VNTRs; 10 to <50 base pairs). There are also other longer, but less common, genetic variations that will not be discussed here. Polymorphisms may fall within coding sequences of genes (exons, so named because they are present in the RNA sequence that is exported out of the nucleus), non-coding regions of genes (introns, so named because they were discovered to be the intervening sequences between exons), or in the intergenic regions (i.e., the regions between genes). In addition, some of these intergenic polymorphisms can occur in segments of DNA adjacent to a gene (flanking regions known as promoters that provide instructions for making RNA from the gene). Compared to within-gene polymorphisms, promoter region polymorphisms are responsible for a large majority of genetic variants associated with phenotypes (Maurano et al., 2012; Nicolae et al., 2010). Although promoter region variants do not result in a protein change, they may play a role in regulating their associated gene. SNPs are the most common type of polymorphism (currently ~10 million known in the human genome) and are the most commonly assessed DNA markers for conducting genetic analyses, particularly when conducting genome-wide association (GWA) studies.

Multiple polymorphisms can also be examined together, for example, through a haplotype. A haplotype is a set of two or more alleles from SNPs that are physically close to each other (linked) on a single chromosome and are inherited together. The alleles present at each SNP result in haplotype patterns that can be evaluated against a target outcome. For example, the *Corticotropin-releasing Hormone Receptor 1* (*CRHR1*) gene has a set of frequently studied alleles at three SNPs: *rs7209436* (T/C), *rs110402* (A/G), and *rs242924* (T/C). The TAT haplotype is the most commonly derived haplotype from these SNPs (e.g., Bradley et al., 2008). Simultaneously examining multiple polymorphisms, such as in haplotypes, allows the analysis of larger portions of the DNA sequence in a single test, which reduces the need for multiple testing. Haplotypes can be identified through public databases and software, such as the 1000 Genomes Project and Haplo Stats 1.4.0, by examining the allele patterns of SNPs.

The high correlation between SNPs that make up a haplotype are characterized in terms of linkage disequilibrium (LD). In general, SNPs that are in close proximity to each other on a chromosome are in high LD. LD can be assessed by a disequilibrium coefficient (D) or the coefficient of correlation (r^2) between SNPs although the latter is preferred by geneticists. LD can be used in GxE research if a new genetic marker becomes of interest, but was not among the variants selected in advance for genotyping. In this case, researchers can overcome not having the SNP among their genotyped variants by using a proxy SNP that is in high LD with the new genetic variant of interest. For example, Cleveland, Griffin, and colleagues, (2018) learned of a genetic variant (*rs6770632*) in the oxytocin receptor (*OXTR*) gene that had been associated with social behavior in a case control study (Malik et al., 2012). This SNP was not genotyped in the Genetics of PROSPER dataset (gPROSPER). Therefore, the research team used a web-based program designed to identify SNPs in linkage disequilibrium, such as SNAP[4] and LDlink,[5] to detect a proxy SNP that was in high linkage disequilibrium (*rs7632287*; $r^2 = 0.95$; 1000 Genomes Project Consortium, 2012) and this proxy SNP was used in place of *rs6770632*.

7.1.1 Quality Control

The ease of large-scale DNA sample collection and genotyping has resulted in much larger genetic datasets, which has led to the need for additional data cleaning and preliminary analyses prior to substantive genotype-phenotype analysis. The initial

---

[4] http://archive.broadinstitute.org/mpg/snap/.

[5] https://analysistools.nci.nih.gov/LDlink/?tab=home.

stages of this process (e.g., data cleaning and checking) require decisions prior to genotyping. First, researchers should include duplicate DNA samples (e.g., ~ five to ten percent of the total sample should be genotyped twice) to check for accuracy once initial genotyping is complete. The amount of duplicate samples researchers need depends on the difficulty of generating the particular genotype due to characteristics of the polymorphism and the technical aspects of the genotyping method, such as pipetting samples into multi-well plates. Staff who conduct genotyping should be blind to which samples are duplicate and duplicates should be removed prior to data analysis. In addition, participants whose DNA genotyping fail at multiple markers (e.g., SNPs, STRs, VNTRs), indicating a high failure rate due to issues with the quality of the DNA sample, should be removed or re-genotyped. Deciding whether to remove a participant or genetic marker can depend on how the genotyping was conducted. For example, when using microarrays to genotype SNPs, a DNA failure rate greater than two to five percent may justify removing participants (Anderson et al., 2010). In contrast, genotyping VNTRs can be more difficult due to the differences in size of the alleles, and what is considered an acceptable error rate can vary, but should generally be no more than five to seven percent. In cases where the re-genotyped results are discrepant from the original genotype results, the participant should be removed from analyses. After this data cleaning process, the overall error rate should be reported in the methods section. Unlike most psychological constructs that contain measurement error, it is possible to assess error magnitude in genotyping measurement using this method.

Following this, the genetic relatedness of participants should be checked through shared alleles that are considered identical by descent (IBD), meaning identifying individuals who possess matching segments of DNA that have been inherited from a recent common ancestor to a greater extent than the general population. Individuals who share a high IBD are more closely genetically related to each other, even if phenotype data does not identify them as biologically related. This method requires analysis of many markers (the number of which depends on the homogeneity of the population being studied) to accurately estimate the IBD relatedness value known as π (which ranges from zero to one); a common strategy is to exclude one individual of a pair with $\pi > 0.2$. It is recommended to randomly remove all but one of each set of biologically related individuals who are closer than third cousins. When the level of relatedness is known, multilevel modeling methods can be used to control for relatedness and allow for the retention of relatives (Wang & Elston, 2005). Thus, if the dataset purposefully has related individuals, this aspect of the design can be addressed statistically.

After participants are removed based on these criteria, the quality of the data should be checked to ensure there are no systematic errors in genotyping, such as mistakenly genotyping the wrong set of samples. First, researchers should check the concordance between self-reported sex and genotype-assessed sex, based on markers on the X and Y chromosomes (an In/Del in the Amelogenin gene can be used; Mannucci, Sullivan, Ivanov, & Gill, 1994). Next, it is important to check whether the genotype frequencies of polymorphisms are consistent with their expected rates found in the general population, known as testing for Hardy–Weinberg equilibrium (HWE). Each allele at a polymorphic site has a frequency, or proportion, of that allele in the population. Most sites contain two alleles and their frequencies are designated with the symbols p and q (where $q = 1 - p$). Pairs of alleles then make genotypes with frequencies of p^2, $2pq$, and q^2. Deviations in HWE can occur due to systematic errors in genotyping, such as an unexpected population structure or the presence of homologous regions in the genome. In some cases, it is common for a specific genetic marker to deviate from HWE and researchers should be careful to identify these instances. Polymorphisms not in HWE should be used with caution because deviation may indicate a genotyping error or sampling bias. In some instances, it may be appropriate to re-genotype participants; however, researchers should also determine if there are instances in the literature of unusual genotype distributions for a specific genetic marker. It is also possible that a polymorphism is not in HWE due to an unusually strong association with the trait being analyzed in a large fraction of the population.

7.2 Brief History of GxE Research

Initially, genetic research focused on studying genetic variants that encoded simple (Mendelian) traits, such as disease, through linkage studies. These studies are of limited value for complex traits that involve multiple interconnected biological pathways and multiple genes working together. The genetic association approach (e.g., candidate gene and GWA studies) has not displaced the linkage approach, but has since emerged as an important tool for studying complex traits. Genetic association analytic methods can concurrently examine many polymorphisms and allow for the study of unrelated individuals, which generates sufficient power to detect polymorphisms that might have small but cumulative effects on specific phenotypes.

The explosion of single candidate gene-by-environment (cGxE) research in behavioral science can be linked to a pair of high-profile studies by Caspi et al. (2002, 2003), the latter leading to considerable debate concerning cGxE research. In this study, Caspi et al. (2003) showed that the serotonin-transporter-linked polymorphic region (*5-HTTLPR*) moderated the association between stressful life events and depression: stressful life events had a larger impact on depression among *5-HTTLPR* short allele carriers, compared to those homozygous for the long allele. These findings were a catalyst for research and discussion on how specific genes may influence the effects of environmental experiences. Subsequent replication attempts of this seminal paper revealed conflicting findings; however, meta-analyses of these replication studies concluded that the *5-HTTLPR* genotype interaction with stressful life events was consistent with chance (Munafò, Durrant, Lewis, & Flint, 2009; Risch et al., 2009; also see Karg, Burmeister, Shedden, & Sen, 2011).

Conclusions offered in these reviews and other commentaries (e.g., Duncan & Keller, 2011) led researchers to question the replicability and validity of all GxE research that uses single markers, whether single-SNPs or candidate genes (Munafò et al., 2009; Risch et al., 2009). Other researchers have found, however, that studies based on datasets with high quality phenotypic measurement had stronger replication records than others (e.g., Rutter, Thapar, & Pickles, 2009). These researchers argued that meta-analytic conclusions were undercut by including large cross-sectional studies with poor measurement, such as long-term retrospective reports, which increases the chance of recall bias, distortions, and inaccuracies (Rutter et al., 2009). Support for the argument that replication problems were linked to study quality, in particular measurement quality, was found by Uher and McGuffin (2010), who determined that *5-HTTLPR* interacted with childhood maltreatment (i.e., stressful life events) to predict persistent depression—but not single episode depression—during adulthood.

This debate is by no means closed. For example, Culverhouse et al. (2017) attempted to address the conflicting finding from multiple meta-analyses to determine the true magnitude of this cGxE finding and the conditions under which it might be observed. The meta-analysis harmonized phenotypes across studies and did not find evidence to support the cGxE hypothesis (Culverhouse et al., 2017). This debate emphasizes the importance of both high quality phenotypic measurement as well as specificity of the phenotype being studied. Both Rutter et al. (2009) and Uher and McGuffin (2008, 2010) concluded that researchers should not discount all cGxE findings, but rather apply more stringent methodological criteria to individual studies. Consistent with their call for careful evaluation of individual studies, below we provide a summary of how to evaluate the quality of individual GxE studies.

Breakout Box 7.1: Focus on Interdisciplinary Work
I have been working in the field of genetics since I was an undergraduate student conducting my thesis on *Drosophila melanogaster* (fruit flies). I have also worked in the field of addiction and neuroimaging. I am now the Research Coordinator for the Laureate Institute for Brain Research's study site of the Adolescent Brain Cognitive Development (ABCD) study funded by the National Institutes of Health. The ABCD study will examine factors that influence brain development in 10,000 children across the United States. Children enroll in the study when they are 9 or 10 years of age and are followed for 10 years. Genetics is an important component of data collection in the ABCD study. During baseline, ABCD will collect genetic data using saliva samples and send the samples to a centralized repository for processing and later analysis. The study of gene and environment interactions is crucially important to understanding risk and resilience factors in development. Genetics allows us to address the nature vs. nurture question, something that has been a goal of scientists for a long time. There are many benefits to studying genetics in behavioral research, but there are also pitfalls. Despite it being easy to collect genetic data, it is very expensive to analyze it, and a lot of genetic data is in storage waiting for funds for analysis. Another challenge that we as researchers need to understand is that genetic findings are not absolute. Findings are complicated, and just because there is a genetic component does not mean that other factors are not involved. That is why it is essential for geneticists to work with behavioral scientists so that they can get the whole picture of development, and answer important questions that can only be answered through interdisciplinary science.

—*Florence Breslin,* MS, CCRP, Manager of Clinical Assessment and Testing

7.3 Evaluating the Quality of GxE Studies

The debate on the validity of cGxE research has led researchers to provide recommendations on how to evaluate GxE studies (see Bakermans-Kranenburg & van Ijzendoorn, 2015; Dick et al., 2015; Salvatore & Dick, 2015; Schlomer, Cleveland, et al., 2015; Uher & McGuffin, 2008). We have synthesized and expanded these recommendations to propose five primary criteria for evaluating the quality of GxE research: (1) study design, (2) theory and statistical methods, (3) controlling for confounds, (4) measurement (phenotype and genotype), and (5) the biological role of polymorphisms. The following sections will elaborate on how GxE research can be evaluated based on these domains and provide examples from previous studies.

7.3.1 Study Design

Study design plays an important role in the ability to detect GxE. Like most behavioral science studies, larger sample sizes are preferred as they increase statistical power for detecting associations (Luan, Wong, Day, & Wareham, 2001). Small sample sizes typical of single gene studies (e.g., $n < 1000$) have been stated as "grossly underpowered" for detecting genetic influences, and research with statistically significant GxE has been charged with leveraging chance results via unreported multiple testing (Dick et al., 2015). The view that candidate gene studies need very large sample sizes stems, in part, from the idea that the effects of any given gene on a phenotype are expected to be quite small based on GWA studies. GWA studies explore thousands to millions of SNPs through bivariate associations with a phenotype. This technique requires a substantial sample size to control for the possibility of detecting an effect due to chance via multiple testing. The effect sizes of bivariate associations found in GWA studies tend to be extremely small, providing support for the assumption that any given SNP will explain only a minuscule amount of variation in a given trait (e.g., Manolio et al., 2009). Given that genetic effects on traits are expected to be small and that interaction terms tend to explain less variance than main effects, it logically follows that larger sample sizes are needed to detect GxE and that previous studies must be underpowered to detect interactions.

The argument that GxE studies need as large or larger sample sizes than GWA studies may not be as straightforward as it seems. The logic supporting the need for huge sample sizes rests on the idea that for every genetic main effect tested in a GWA study, a corresponding GxE term also needs to be tested, effectively doubling the number of associations when a single environment is evaluated. In genetic analyses that target a homogeneous environmental experience, sample sizes of this magnitude would not be needed. Further, GxE research assumes, unlike GWA studies, that genetic associations are not uniform across environments (e.g., there may be a larger effect in a disadvantaged neighborhood than in an advantaged neighborhood) or subpopulations (e.g., there may be a larger effect in African compared to European ancestry populations exposed to an environment; Schlomer et al., 2017). As a result, the overall genetic main effect of any given SNP may be small and difficult to detect statistically when the study sample captures and averages over multiple environmental contexts, developmental periods, and/or populations. Thus, increasing power via increased sample size alone may have the net effect of limiting (or even reducing) the detectable genetic effect size due to increasing contextual and/or ancestral heterogeneity (Schlomer, Fosco, Cleveland, Vandenbergh, & Feinberg, 2015; Schlomer et al., 2017). Under the right conditions, such as focusing on a specific developmental context and population, using well-measured constructs, GxE researchers should be able to detect genetic main effects and/or interactions with smaller sample sizes.

An additional challenge of GxE research is that, like most studies, GxE studies can be confounded by the presence of gene-environment correlation (*r*GE). Environments are not randomly assigned to individuals, rather environmental conditions are correlated with individuals' genetic predispositions through different processes (e.g., *passive, active,* and *evocative r*GE*;* see Scarr & McCartney, 1983). For example, the correlation between positive parenting and adolescent substance use may reflect a passive *r*GE whereby genes shared by parent and child contribute to both positive parenting and lower substance use. Genetically influenced characteristics may account for environmental reactions to individuals (evocative *r*GE) and/or result in individuals selecting environments that suit their genetic dispositions (active *r*GE). Randomized intervention and experimental designs eliminate passive and active *r*GE with respect to the manipulation because researchers choose which environmental condition participants experience (e.g., Creswell et al., 2012; Larsen et al., 2010). Randomized designs can also increase statistical power through more precise measurement of the environment (e.g., intervention/control), and the number of participants needed to obtain the same statistical power as correlational GxE studies is decreased through randomization (McClelland & Judd, 1993). Correlational studies can attempt to control for *r*GE through preliminary analyses that determine whether the specific genetic variant is associated with the study's environmental variables (e.g., Janssens et al., 2015). This statistical approach is limited, as it does not address whether the key environmental variables are correlated with other genetic variants not investigated. Thus, any GxE finding may be due to an unmeasured *r*GE that is correlated with both the gene and the environment under investigation.

7.3.2 Theory and Statistical Methods

A major strength of behavioral and developmental research is the use of theories to guide hypotheses that frame decisions about which environments and phenotypes to examine, how to operationalize and measure constructs, and what population(s) to examine. These strengths lend themselves well to GxE research because the selection of the gene, environment, and phenotype are critical to the validity of GxE findings. For example, Schlomer, Fosco, et al. (2015) drew on existing research on the Cognitive-Contextual Framework (Fosco, DeBoard, & Grych, 2007) to develop a model of individual differences in adolescent internalizing problems. The framework pointed to specific aspects of the environment and developmental outcome that were then tested with a GxE approach. Schlomer, Fosco, et al. (2015) found that processes linking interparental conflict with adolescent internalizing problems—as stipulated by the Cognitive Contextual Framework—differed depending on *DRD4* genotype.

Using theory to inform GxE studies can help researchers avoid multiple testing by narrowing the research space (i.e., theory can limit the set of constructs and environments examined). In addition, compared to an exploratory approach, theory can increase the *a priori* probability that a detected GxE is not a false positive via hypothesis-driven analyses. Lastly, theory and biological knowledge can be useful for determining which gene(s) should be studied in conjunction with the phenotype and environment, particularly when the theory postulates specific intra-individual and/or biological processes (Schlomer & Cho, 2017).

An important developmental theory relevant to GxE research is the risk and resilience framework. Studies guided by this framework have used statistical moderation to investigate risk and protective factors that moderate the impact of adversity on development (Luthar et al., 2000; Masten, 2001). This framework and statistical method has been interpreted by some to assume that the shape of the interaction should conform to the diathesis stress model where adversity leads to maladjustment among some individuals while resilient individuals are unaffected (Monroe & Simons, 1991). Diathesis stress, or inherent stress sensitivities, posits that environmental conditions can act as a trigger, such that the presence of specific environmental contexts (e.g., child maltreatment) exacerbates an inherited propensity for a specific outcome (e.g., depression; Monroe & Simons, 1991). When applied to GxE research, this framework leads to the proposition that the effects of environmental contexts are intensified by some individuals' genetic liability, which results in heterogeneous developmental outcomes. Conversely, in the absence of environmental triggers or in the presence of an enriching environment, differences in genetic liability toward maladaptive outcomes are not observed.

Much of the more recent GxE research has been guided by Differential Susceptibility Theory (DST; Belsky et al., 2007; Belsky & Pluess, 2009; Ellis, Boyce, Belsky, Bakermans-Kranenburg, & van Ijzendoorn, 2011). Based on evolutionary theory, DST augments the diathesis stress model by further positing that the same characteristics that may make an individual vulnerable to adversity may confer a significant advantage under more favorable circumstances. Accordingly, individuals do not possess a propensity toward maladaptive outcomes, but rather a sensitivity to both adverse and favorable environments (Belsky et al., 2007; Belsky & Pluess, 2009; Ellis et al., 2011). In adverse environments, individuals with low environmental sensitivity are less affected by the adverse experiences. In contrast, individuals with high environmental sensitivity are more affected. As such, individuals with low inherited sensitivity to environments are also less positively affected by favorable environments, and those with high environmental sensitivity tend to flourish under these conditions.

Individuals' responses to environmental conditions, either consistent with diathesis stress or DST, have implications for the expected shape of the statistical interaction: fan shaped for diathesis-stress and cross-over for DST (Roisman et al., 2012). Early GxE researchers drew conclusions about interaction forms by visually inspecting the interaction shape. More recently, methodological recommendations have been made to more rigorously examine interactions, such as calculating the regions of significance (Aiken & West, 1991; Preacher, Curran, & Bauer, 2006), the standard error of the interaction cross-over point (Widaman et al., 2012), and the proportion of the interaction index and proportion of affected index (Roisman et al., 2012). Empirically evaluating the shape of the GxE allows researchers to more rigorously interpret whether findings are in support of diathesis-stress or DST models and at what point or under what conditions individuals begin to differ in their environmental response (Reiss, Leve, & Neiderhiser, 2013; Roisman et al., 2012; Villafuerte, Trucco, Heitzeg, Burmeister, & Zucker, 2014). In order for these statistical tests to have implications for underlying theories, it is critical that both favorable and adverse environmental contexts, as well as positive and negative behavioral outcomes, be sampled and measured.

7.3.3 Controlling for Confounds

Failure to control for potential confounds (e.g., gender, ethnicity, and socioeconomic status) can create problems in any study, but there are unique challenges when taking confounds into account when conducting GxE research. GxE studies must control for genetic ancestry, as allele frequencies may vary by populations with distinguishable genetic ancestry backgrounds. Population stratification (i.e., allelic associations due to systematic differences in genetic ancestry, also known as population structure) can result in allele frequencies differing between ancestral populations (Freedman et al., 2004). When allele frequencies differ across populations and the target outcome is correlated with ancestry, results may be spurious due to allelic differences across ancestral populations driving the association. Studies can address this issue by analyzing ancestry subgroups separately, eliminating sparse ancestry groups from the sample, and using ancestry informative genetic markers (AIMs) as a statistical control. Of these methods, controlling for allelic differences across ancestral populations using AIMs is best, however, a less ideal alternative would be to limit analyses to homogenous ancestral groups.

AIMs are SNPs that have different genotype frequencies dependent on the geographical region from which the population originates and provide one method that can be used to address population stratification (Halder, Shriver, Thomas, Fernandez, & Frudakis, 2008). AIMs are first used to generate a matrix of pairwise allele-sharing distances among all pairs in the sample, which can be done with the commonly used PLINK 1.9 software (see Purcell et al., 2007). Principal coordinates

(PC) analysis is then performed on the distance matrix to generate PCs. Biplots of the PCs represent the major axes of genetic variation in the sample and can be merged with self-reported ancestry to visualize the axis of genetic variation represented by each PC. The number of AIMs needed for PC analysis varies by the ancestry of the sample, but successful analyses have used as few as 34 (Cleveland, Griffin, et al., 2018; Cleveland, Schlomer, et al., 2018). This approach, however, varies in usefulness across ancestral groupings. Ancestral groupings with more genetic admixture, such as Hispanics, have a population structure more difficult to identify.

For example, Cleveland et al. (2015) used this technique in a GxE study to control for population stratification by including it as a covariate in regression models. In their sample, two PCs captured a large portion of the variability in allele-sharing distances; PC1 accounted for approximately 10% and PC2 accounted for 6%. Biplots of population structure combined with self-reported ethnicity indicated that PC1 indexed non-European ancestry (e.g., self-reported African Americans and Hispanics), while PC2 indexed the difference between African Americans and Hispanics. In a sample of 555 participants, PC1 classified 507 as having European ancestry and 48 as having non-European ancestry. The genetically informed classification identified 6 of 7 individuals who self-reported as African American, 26 of 27 who self-reported as Hispanic, 3 of 4 who self-reported as Asian, and 2 self-reported Whites as having non-European ancestry. It is important to note, however, that a key aspect of controlling for population stratification is that the specific solutions needed are driven by the ancestral characteristics and distribution of the analytic sample.

7.3.4 Measurement

Phenotypic and genotypic measurement is equally important to rigorously examining a GxE. As previously mentioned, poor phenotypic measurement may explain the inability to replicate studies because it reduces power to detect GxE (Bakermans-Kranenburg & van Ijzendoorn, 2015; Dick et al., 2015; Manuck & McCaffery, 2014; Monroe & Reid, 2008; Schlomer, Cleveland, et al., 2015; Schlomer, Fosco, et al., 2015; Uher & McGuffin, 2008; van Ijzendoorn et al., 2011). Poor measurement introduces random error that otherwise limits the detectable effect size because the ratio of true construct variance to error variance is lower. When phenotypic measurement is poor and genotypic measurement is reliable, there is an increased risk for both Type I and Type II errors because of divergent error variations (Bakermans-Kranenburg & van Ijzendoorn, 2015; van Ijzendoorn et al., 2011).

Evaluating the phenotypic measurement in a study requires considering numerous aspects. For example, prospective measurement is preferred over retrospective measurement, particularly in research that investigates developmental processes. As demonstrated by Caspi et al. (2003), prospective and retrospective measurement can play an important role in detecting GxE by reducing recall bias and measurement error. Another important factor for measurement quality involves the measurement instrument and the reporter. Phenotypes must be measured using developmentally meaningful assessments to ensure construct validity. For example, Caspi et al. (2003) assessed depression with multiple meaningfully equivalent measures of depression including depressive symptoms, major depressive episodes, and suicide attempts. Constructs must be assessed with reporters (i.e., observational task, teacher-, parent-, or self-report) best able to quantify the phenomenon of interest. In addition, the use of multiple reports, whether it is self-, parent-, teacher-report, and/or clinically assessed, can help reduce same-source bias, thereby increasing the detection of a reliable GxE. In addition, how measures are scaled also plays an important role in measurement quality. For example, the full range of responses on a continuous variable should be used rather than artificially dichotomizing (e.g., median split). Dichotomizing continuous variables restricts the range of the variable and limits construct variance, which can thereby reduce the ability to detect GxE effects.

The quality of genotypic measurement requires knowledge of how specific genetic variants are coded. Studies designate the "risk" allele or genotype that affects the functionality of the polymorphisms and how the functionality relates to the phenotype of interest. For example, the *Dopamine Receptor D4* (*DRD4*) gene contains a VNTR that is often coded based on the presence or absence of the 7-repeat allele because this allele is associated with altered gene expression (Schoots & Van Tol, 2003) and diminished concentration-dependent inhibition of forskolin-stimulated cyclicAMP (cAMP) levels (Asghari et al., 1995). When the functional effect of the "risk" allele is known, genotypes can be coded to reflect an additive effect (i.e., cumulative effect of "active" allele; 0/1/2), dominant effect (i.e., "active" allele expression prohibits the expression of the other allele; 0/1), or recessive effect ("active" allele requires two copies to be active; 0/1). As another example, the *Catechol-O-methyltransferase* (*COMT*) gene has a valine (Val) to methionine (Met) mutation, such that the Met allele codes for an enzyme that decreases dopamine catabolism, compared with the enzyme that is coded by the Val allele (Chen et al., 2004), and increased ventral striatum reactivity (Yacubian et al., 2007). Variation in the *COMT* gene has been shown to function additively, meaning each Met allele is associated with increased dopamine production (Val/Val = 0, Val/Met = 1, Met/Met = 2; Chen et al., 2004). It is important to note that if there are too few minor allele homozygous individuals, possibly due to examining a rare polymorphism and/or small sample size, the additive method will be limited. One solution to this issue has been to combine the rare homozygotes with heterozygotes (i.e., assuming a dominance effect) to increase statistical power. Although this method provides a statistical advantage, researchers should evaluate how the coding scheme relates to genetic function as well as the subsequent meaning of their findings.

For some polymorphisms, how the "risk" allele operates is not known. This ambiguity can be addressed with planned comparisons of each genotype. For example, dummy codes can be used to capture the interactive effects of a gene without constraining a model to be linear, and utilizes two cross-product terms (see Aliev, Latendresse, Bacanu, Neale, and Dick (2014) for a related approach). The dummy codes are simultaneously tested within the same model with two main effect variables and two interaction terms. If both interaction terms are significant, there is evidence of an additive genetic effect. Alternatively, if only one interaction term is significant, there is evidence of a dominant or recessive genetic effect (Aliev et al., 2014).

7.3.5 Biological Role of Genes

It is also critical to consider whether a GxE study is guided by how the genetic variant may be biologically linked to the examined phenotype. A great deal of cG×E studies, especially early research, relied on a handful of "usual suspect" candidate genes (Munafò, 2006; e.g., *SLC6A4*, *MAOA*, *DRD4*) and some have argued that these variants are used in contexts where there is not a clear biological connection between the gene and the phenotype. Since this early work, researchers have expanded the scope of GxE work beyond the "usual suspects" by considering how genetic variants linked to specific biological processes lead to variation in phenotypes related to these biological processes. For example, Vandenbergh and colleagues (2015) selected five polymorphisms (*rs1948*, *rs578776*, *rs588765*, *rs684513*, and *rs16969968*) in a set of nicotinic acetylcholine receptor subunit genes (*CHRNA5*/*A3*/*B4*) in close proximity to one another and related to tobacco use. These markers were identified through prior work on genomic function, research using haplotypes, and GWA studies (see Vandenbergh & Schlomer, 2014). For example, the *rs16969968* polymorphism within the fifth exon of *CHRNA5* gene is part of a haplotype that moderated the effects of a drug treatment to predict cessation (Chen et al., 2012) as well as being identified in a GWAS-polygenic risk score that moderated the effects of randomized drug therapy (Uhl et al., 2010, 2014). The other markers in this set were included because they had been associated with some smoking-related phenotypes in other studies (Stephens et al., 2013) and their inclusion allowed assessment of the entire region of interest in these three genes, rather than just analyzing the effect of *rs16969968* and the DNA in LD with it.

Early cGxE work began with "usual suspect" candidate genes (Munafò, 2006) largely because prior to high density genotyping, this small set of genes had been a major focus of research in other disciplines (e.g., mouse studies) and much was already known about them. However, the literature has since expanded as a result of new technologies to incorporating different genetic variants beyond this small set of genes. These developments represent a crossroad of how behavioral scientists might continue to incorporate "usual suspect" genes into their studies. On the one hand, the "usual suspects" might be relevant. In fact, a good deal of the evolutionarily inspired DST research has used these genes with some success. On the other hand, there is no reason to believe that these genes are critical for all outcomes. Analyzing associations between these usual suspects and outcomes need to be supported by strong arguments linking the genetic variation to the phenotype, or in the case of GxE, linking the genetic variation to sensitivity to the particular aspect of the environment being studied; however, to the extent that the phenotype is well-studied within the animal literature and there is an understanding of how specific genes influence biological processes linked to the phenotype, there appear to be many opportunities still for behavioral scientists to incorporate other candidate genes into their analyses.

7.4 Polygenic Scores: Next Wave of Genetic Variance Assessments

Although studying a single gene or genetic marker is justified when its biological function is well-understood and lends insight into mechanisms of gene-phenotype links, it is also clear that complex traits of interest to behavioral scientists are regulated by multiple genes (Turkheimer, 2000). Concerns over the latter has led to the critique that cGxE research overly relies on studies that use only one genetic variant (i.e., using only one gene or one SNP). One way this criticism has been addressed is by aggregating multiple genetic variants into a polygenic score. Depending on the specific genetic variants used to create the composite, different terms have been used, such as "gene score," "SNP score," or "multi-locus genetic profile." Testing the effects of multiple genetic markers in and around genetic areas of interest via gene scores diminishes multiple testing problems that occur when multiple candidate genes are individually tested within the same study or in GWA studies that test the association between many thousands of genetic variants with a single trait. The sections below explain two approaches to creating these genetic scores: biologically based and data driven.

7.4.1 Biologically Based Polygenic Scores

Biologically based polygenic scores are derived from genes relevant to physiologic functions such as neurotransmitters (e.g., dopamine and serotonin) or biochemical pathways. Biologically based polygenetic scores usually include only a few polymorphisms linked to the receptors or metabolic enzymes related to the neurotransmitter or pathway of interest; rarely are all possible polymorphisms included in these scores. Polygenic scores can include multiple polymorphisms in different genes related to the same neurotransmitter system, multiple SNPs in a single gene, multiple polymorphisms related to a biochemical pathway, multiple polymorphisms in multiple genes that span different neurotransmitter systems, or based on the biologically relevant gene function.

In a score composed of polymorphisms in multiple genes within the same neurotransmitter system, each incorporated gene should play a functional role relevant to the neurotransmitter system. For example, multiple dopaminergic polymorphisms are likely to shape variability in brain function. Nikolova, Ferrell, Manuck, and

Hariri (2011) used a positive and negative feedback task to engage ventral striatum reactivity to test whether individual differences in ventral striatum reactivity responsiveness were associated with genetic differences. A multilocus genetic profile aggregated five sites of genetic variation in four genes [*DAT1*, *DRD4*, *DRD2* (−141C In/ Del and Taq1A), and *COMT*] to capture variability in dopamine neurotransmitter signaling. This score explained 10.9% of the individual differences in ventral striatum dopamine signaling during the task (Nikolova et al., 2011).

In addition to variability across multiple genes, a single gene can contain multiple genetic variants (e.g., SNPs). Genetic variants within a gene may be closely related and thereby constitute the same genetic variation (e.g., SNPs in high linkage equilibrium) or each SNP may uniquely affect the functionality of a gene (e.g., SNPs in low linkage disequilibrium). Multiple SNPs within a gene, in either high or low LD, can be aggregated to make a biologically based polygenic score. Cleveland, Griffin, and colleagues (2018) identified five SNPs (*rs6770632*, *rs53576*, *rs2254298*, *rs4686302*, and *rs1488467*) in the *OXTR* gene in low linkage disequilibrium that capture unique variation in the oxytocin receptor, which encodes for the receptor protein regulating oxytocin signaling during social interactions. SNPs were coded based on prior findings and aggregated to create a multi-SNP single-gene index of variation in the *OXTR* gene, in which higher values on the *OXTR* score indicated increased sensitivity to social interactions. Cleveland, Griffin, and colleagues (2018) examined whether the *OXTR* gene score moderated the associations between a substance use preventative intervention (intervention vs. control), target adolescent-nominated peer substance use, and early adolescent alcohol use. A primary finding of this study was that low *OXTR* gene score values were linked to affiliating with friends who reported less substance use in the intervention condition compared to the control condition.

In contrast to scores based on a set of genes related to a neurotransmitter system, a biochemical pathway polygenic score is composed of genetic polymorphisms that capture the steps of a metabolic pathway. A biochemical pathway is a chain of chemical reactions catalyzed by enzymes that either synthesize or break down molecules, such as the chemical reactions needed to metabolize alcohol. The body metabolizes alcohol through a two-step biochemical pathway: (1) alcohol dehydrogenase enzymes (ADH) metabolize alcohol to acetaldehyde and (2) acetaldehyde is further metabolized into acetate (Zakhari, 2006). Research has shown that a number of polymorphisms in ADH genes affect ADH enzymes that are important to alcohol metabolism (processing ethanol to acetaldehyde; reviewed by Edenberg & Foroud, 2014). For example, the *ADH1B* gene contains a SNP (*rs1229984*) whose major allele results in a slower rate of alcohol oxidation into acetaldehyde, which slows alcohol metabolism. Slower alcohol metabolism increases the concentration of alcohol in the body, resulting in inebriation, and diminishes the concentration of acetaldehyde.

Cleveland, Schlomer, et al. (2018) simultaneously tested the effects of three SNP scores for three alcohol dehydrogenase genes, *ADH1B* (*rs1042026* and *rs1229984*), *ADH1C* (*rs698* and *rs1614972*), and *ADH4* (*rs1126671* and *rs1800759*). The two markers for each gene were aggregated such that higher values correspond to greater alcohol use risk. The *ADH1B* and *ADH1C* scores significantly predicted ninth grade alcohol use and change in early-to-mid adolescent alcohol use. The association between *ADH1C* and alcohol use (both intercept and slope) was reduced when individuals were in the intervention condition.

Finally, it is also possible for polygenic scores to be composed of polymorphisms from multiple genes within different neurotransmitter systems. Combining the effects of polymorphisms across neurotransmitter systems is justifiable when studies demonstrate that the two systems interact with one another, or when the different genes are known to be related to the same trait of interest. For example, although dopamine and serotonin are two different neurotransmitters, the distinct dopaminergic and serotonergic systems have been shown to have strong anatomical and functional interactions with each other (Kapur & Remington, 1996) and are theorized to be reciprocal (Daw, Kakade, & Dayan, 2002; Wong, Feng, & Teo, 1995). Belsky and Beaver (2011) used an across-system score that aggregated genetic variants across multiple genes associated with dopaminergic and/or serotonergic system function hypothesized to increase environmental sensitivity (i.e., *DAT1*, DRD2, *DRD4*, *5-HTTLPR*, and *MAOA)*. Polymorphisms were coded to reflect higher levels of environmental sensitivity to create a cumulative index. In this study, cumulative genetic sensitivity and both supportive and unsupportive parenting had differential effects on self-regulation. Males with more sensitive alleles were more effected by supportive and unsupportive parenting, resulting in the more and less self-regulation (Belsky & Beaver, 2011).

7.4.2 Data-Driven Polygenic Scores

In contrast to biologically based approaches, data-driven approaches to polygenic scores use results from a GWA study to create a score. The top “hits” from a GWA study conducted on a target phenotype are aggregated together to form a genetic score that is then used in an independent dataset to predict the same phenotype or similar phenotypes. Choosing SNPs to be included in the score typically follows a two-step process. First, the GWA study is conducted on a discovery sample to test the relationship between individual SNPs and a target trait. The SNPs most strongly associated with a trait (e.g., the top five percent of SNPs with the lowest p values) are weighted based on their univariate association with the trait. Second, in a new sample with similar data, SNPs identified from the discovery sample, or proxy SNPs, are combined into a weighted sum to produce an aggregate SNP score for each person. The score is then used to predict the trait of interest within the new sample. Unlike biologically based approaches, this approach is indifferent to the genomic function of the genetic markers that make up the score.

Musci et al. (2015) examined whether a genome-wide polygenic score and an intervention was associated with first tobacco use. A GWA study was conducted on randomized smoking cessation trial in a sample of smoking adults to identify genetic variants associated with successfully quitting smoking (Uhl et al., 2010). Twelve thousands SNPs were included in the score based on their significant association (i.e., $p < .01$) with successful cessation of smoking. Scores were weighted based on strength and replicability of SNP associations, which resulted in a continuous variable with higher scores indicating more alleles across SNPs associated with greater success in smoking cessation. Participants at the higher end of the polygenic score benefitted the most from the intervention in terms of delayed age of first use (Musci et al., 2015). Although GWAS-derived gene scores can explain more variance in a phenotype than a single SNP, or group of SNPs, behavioral researchers may not have the resources to conduct their own GWA study. Instead, researchers can use existing GWA studies to inform their polygenetic scores (see Belsky et al., 2013).

7.5 Implications

7.5.1 Implications for Understanding Family Resilience

The risk and resilience framework requires individuals to demonstrate resilience by overcoming the effects of adversity and achieving successful development (Luthar & Zigler, 1991; Masten, Best, & Garmezy, 1990; Rutter, 1987). Adversity affects individuals differently, and resilience is not always achieved. This observation begs the question "*What factors explain individual differences in responses to adversity?*" Factors identified in prior research include individual characteristics (e.g., parent personality), aspects of the family relationship (e.g., marital conflict), and environmental features (e.g., economic strain, social support network; reviewed in, Black & Lobo, 2008). Biological factors, such as genetics, need to be added to this list. Not only is their consideration important to fully understanding the process of resilience, failure to account for these influences can inflate the perception that only environmental influences impact the development of resilience. For example, genetic variance may underlie how family members respond to adversity and be linked to the family environment that effect resilience (Cicchetti, 2010; Egeland et al., 1993; Luthar et al., 2000). Thus, it is important to provide resilience researchers the tools to investigate the impact of genetic differences, to understand the extent that genetic influences and family environments impact resilience.

Integrating GxE approaches with family resilience research opens the way to new questions that can be asked and evaluated. The plethora of research on family resilience is a considerable strength, as this research serves as a foundation that could be built on by genetically informed research. For example, how families and family members respond to adversity, and demonstrate resilience, may be influenced by genetic sensitivity to the environment. Genetic variations may play a role in how risk and protective characteristics impact family resilience. Integrating GxE approaches to investigate questions such as these can examine underlying genetic mechanisms that may be linked to individual differences in resilience responses within the family system. This integration will provide an important tool for considering how some families overcome adverse environments as well as help explain why individuals in the same families, such as siblings, can differ considerably in resilience.

The theoretical frameworks that guide family resilience research can be used to inform research questions and hypotheses when genetic mechanisms are incorporated. Theoretical frameworks and previous evidence can guide researchers to the most pertinent environments and phenotypes to examine and how to operationalize and measure relevant constructs. For example, the deviance proneness model proposes that children of substance-abusing parents inherit a genetic predisposition for impulsivity that may be associated with substance use (Iacono, Malone, & McGue, 2008). To build on this framework, Elam et al. (2016) examined bidirectional transactions between children's impulsivity and family conflict and their later substance use while incorporating the impact of mothers', fathers', and children's polygenic risk scores. Combined phenotypic and genetic data from multiple family members (e.g., mother-, father-, and child-report) can then be used to examine parent- and child-driven genetic influences as well as whether there is an intergenerational transmission of genetic sensitivity. For example, Elam et al. (2017) examined whether children's elevated polygenetic risk impacted impulsivity in middle childhood, and whether children's biologically influenced impulsivity evoked family conflict later in childhood. By integrating a GxE approach with a theoretical framework, researchers can investigate biological mechanisms previously only theorized to impact family systems.

7.5.2 Implications for Policy

Behavioral genetic designs have provided foundational evidence that there are heritable influences on complex behavioral traits (Turkheimer, 2000) and that heritable influences can be modified by environmental experiences (Leve, Harold, Ge, Neiderhiser, & Patterson, 2010; Reiss & Leve, 2007). Furthering this body of work, molecular genetic GxE and gene-by-environment intervention (GxI) research has provided evidence that genetic variations modify the effects of environments and interventions (e.g., Beach, Brody, Lei, and Philibert, 2010, b; Brody, Beach, Philibert, Chen, Lei, Murry, and Brown, 2009; Brody, Beach, Philibert, Chen, and Murry, 2009; Cleveland et al., 2015). The potential implications for policy and prevention based on molecular genetic research are only theoretical because the molecular genetic GxE literature is relatively young, starting in the early 2000s. Researchers are just beginning to identify environmental contexts that reduce or exacerbate how genes and interventions interact (e.g., Cleveland, Griffin et al., 2018; Cleveland et al., 2015), developmental time periods when genes are more impactful (e.g., Russell et al., 2018), and different types and dosages of interventions that interact with genes (e.g., Howe, Beach, & Brody, 2010). Prior to translating GxE and GxI findings to prevention and policy efforts, the literature needs to increase the sophistication with which it operationalizes genetic variance. Not only does the field need to move past single-gene operationalization of genetic influences, but the field must also move past simplistic main effects conceptualizations of how genes act that underlie most GWA investigations.

A central focus of this chapter is emphasizing the value in moving beyond examining a single candidate gene to examining the impact of multiple genetic variants that operate in concert through polygenic risk scores. Polygenic scores are able to index the impact of multiple genetic variants to investigate their combined impact on complex traits, known to be influenced by multiple genes. Polygenic approaches are a promising avenue to investigate GxE and GxI effects, and the combination of genes that might influence complex traits has not been exhausted. Rather, researchers have barely scratched the surface of the possible ways in which genes might operate together and influence development, with multiple genes and with environments. In addition, as genotyping technology advances, researchers will be better able to conceptualize and operationalize genetic variance.

Researchers have begun to theorize about the potential implications of molecular genetic research for policy and prevention (e.g., Belsky & van Ijzendoorn, 2015; Cleveland, Schlomer, Vandenbergh, & Wiebe, 2016; Gajos, Fagan, & Beaver, 2016; Musci & Schlomer, 2017). Two approaches for translating evidence from genetically informed designs to prevention programs and policy have been set forth. One approach suggests that evidence from genetically informed designs should be used to allocate prevention and public-health resources to the most sensitive populations based on individual's genetic vulnerability or plasticity (Belsky, 2014; Gajos, Fagan, & Beaver, 2016). Another approach suggests that when genetically informed designs identify individuals who are not benefiting from current prevention efforts, more resources should be devoted to developing the type and dosage of interventions that will help those who need more assistance (Cleveland et al., 2016). Building on these approaches, we propose that information from genetically informed designs should be added to improve how prevention programs are implemented, such as the use of adaptive intervention programs that take into account how individuals respond to programs (see Collins, Murphy, & Strecher, 2007). GxE and GxI studies can potentially be used to identify the minimum dosage needed for each intervention so fewer resources are allocated toward individuals already benefiting from prevention programs and more resources can be directed toward less responsive individuals who still need assistance.

Due to the fact that GxE and GxI research is still in its infancy, current evidence needs to be replicated and extended to different populations (e.g., ethnic groups and socioeconomic statuses). GxE and GxI research necessitates that genetic influences differ by environmental conditions, meaning that findings are sensitive to children's developmental period, and the type of intervention being used. In addition, with notable exceptions (see Beach, Brody, Lei, & Philibert, 2010; Brody, Beach, Philibert, Chen, & Murry, 2009), GxE and GxI research has primarily studied individuals of European ancestry from financially secure backgrounds (e.g., middle to upper-middle class; Fullerton, Yu, Crouch, Fryer-Edwards, & Burke, 2010; Knerr, Wayman, & Bonham, 2011). Thus, not only is it important to understand how GxE processes apply across environmental and developmental contexts, researchers must also investigate the extent to which GxE findings can be generalized to other populations prior to being used to shape policy and prevention efforts.

7.6 Conclusion

A central assumption of the risk and resilience framework is that individuals vary in their response to environmental experiences. GxE research has become an increasingly popular and valuable approach to examining biological sensitivity that leads individuals to vary in response to environmental experiences. Although it is widely accepted that both genetic and environmental factors contribute to development, rarely has risk and resilience research taken the role of genetic influences into account. GxE research advances our understanding of development by examining how genes and environmental experiences interact with each other to contribute to a wide variety of complex behavioral outcomes. This chapter has provided a brief overview of molecular genetics, genetic data quality control checks, cGxE research and its criticisms, and a framework for evaluating the quality of GxE studies. The overview culminates in ways polygenic scores can measure genetic variance and can be used by behavioral scientists to advance GxE research.

We encourage behavioral scientists interested in investigating GxE association to begin considering strategies for adding genotypic data to their own studies of risk and resilience. Incorporating molecular genetic data into behavioral science provides opportunities to advance our understanding of how GxE transactions influence resilience processes. This type of research, however, is an interdisciplinary endeavor that requires collaborations between multiple fields (e.g., molecular genetics, psychology, and statistics). We encourage behavioral scientists to reach across these fields and build the mutually beneficial collaborative research groups necessary to develop and execute studies that are both innovative and protected from the challenges outlined.

Regardless of topic or field, high quality research requires that many different threats to validity be addressed. The primary goal of this chapter was to set out methodological challenges that confront GxE research and introduce the reader to strategies for how these threats can be addressed. Our list of challenges research should consider includes study design, theoretical approach, statistical method, controls for population stratification, phenotype and genotype measurement, and the biological role of polymorphisms. This list is not meant to be exhaustive, but rather, aims to provide researchers who are new to GxE research a starting point when they begin to design their own GxE studies. Behavioral scientists' focus on developmental processes and measurement of contexts and experiences positions them with the ability to make important contributions to GxE research. Fulfilling this potential, however, will require that they develop research projects that address the specific threats that can otherwise undercut the validity of their research findings.

Discussion Questions

1. A major strength of integrating behavior and developmental research with GxE designs are the theories behavioral scientists use to guide hypotheses. Select and define a theory relevant to your research and explain how a GxE design could be used to investigate core components of the selected theory.

2. Develop a research question, design, and hypothesis that could be examined within a GxE design. Provide detailed information on how constructs will be operationalized, the biological importance of the selected genetic variation, and how the genetic variation will modify environmental experiences.
3. Select a published GxE study relevant to your research interests. Summarize the study's theoretical approach, the theorized biological role of the genetic variation, measurement (phenotype and genotype), statistical method, and the ability to control for confounds. Evaluate the study based on these domains and identify how you would improve the quality of the study.

References

1000 Genomes Project Consortium. (2012). An integrated map of genetic variation from 1,092 human genomes. *Nature, 491*(7422), 56–65. https://doi.org/10.1038/nature11632

Aiken, L., & West, S. (1991). *Multiple regression: Testing and interpreting interactions*. Thousand Oaks, CA: Sage.

Aliev, F., Latendresse, S. J., Bacanu, S. A., Neale, M. C., & Dick, D. M. (2014). Testing for measured gene-environment interaction: Problems with the use of cross-product terms and a regression model reparameterization solution. *Behavior Genetics, 44*(2), 165–181. https://doi.org/10.1007/s10519-014-9642-1

Anderson, C. A., Pettersson, F. H., Clarke, G. M., Cardon, L. R., Morris, A. P., & Zondervan, K. T. (2010). Data quality control in genetic case-control association studies. *Nature Protocols, 5*(9), 1564–1573. https://doi.org/10.1038/nprot.2010.116

Asghari, V., Sanyal, S., Buchwaldt, S., Paterson, A., Jovanovic, V., & Van Tol, H. H. (1995). Modulation of intracellular cyclic AMP levels by different human dopamine D4 receptor variants. *Journal of Neurochemistry, 65*(3), 1157–1165. https://doi.org/10.1046/j.1471-4159.1995.65031157.x

Ayorech, Z., Selzam, S., Smith-Woolley, E., Knopik, V. S., Neiderhiser, J. M., DeFries, J. C., & Plomin, R. (2016). Publication trends over 55 years of behavioral genetic research. *Behavior Genetics, 46*(5), 603–607. https://doi.org/10.1007/s10519-016-9786-2

Bakermans-Kranenburg, M. J., & van Ijzendoorn, M. H. (2015). The hidden efficacy of interventions: Gene×environment experiments from a differential susceptibility perspective. *Annual Review of Psychology, 66*(1), 381–409. https://doi.org/10.1146/annurev-psych-010814-015407

Beach, S. R. H., Brody, G. H., Lei, M.-K., & Philibert, R. A. (2010). Differential susceptibility to parenting among African American youths: Testing the DRD4 hypothesis. *Journal of Family Psychology, 24*(5), 513–521. https://doi.org/10.1037/a0020835

Belsky, D. W., Moffitt, T. E., Baker, T. B., Biddle, A. K., Evans, J. P., Harrington, H., … Caspi, A. (2013). Polygenic risk and the developmental progression to heavy, persistent smoking and nicotine dependence: Evidence from a 4-decade longitudinal study. *JAMA Psychiatry, 70*(5), 534–542. https://doi.org/10.1001/jamapsychiatry.2013.736

Belsky, J. (2014, November 30). The downside of resilience. *New York Times*, p. 34.

Belsky, J., Bakermans-kranenburg, M. J., Van Ijzendoorn, M. H., Issues, S., Kingdom, U., & Studies, F. (2007). For better and for worse: Differential susceptibility to environmental influences. *Current Directions in Psychological Science, 16*(6), 300–304. https://doi.org/10.1111/j.1467-8721.2007.00525.x

Belsky, J., & Beaver, K. M. (2011). Cumulative-genetic plasticity, parenting and adolescent self-regulation. *Journal of Child Psychology and Psychiatry, 52*(5), 619–626. https://doi.org/10.1111/j.1469-7610.2010.02327.x

Belsky, J., & Pluess, M. (2009). Beyond diathesis stress: Differential susceptibility to environmental influences. *Psychological Bulletin, 135*(6), 885–908. https://doi.org/10.1037/a0017376

Belsky, J., & van Ijzendoorn, M. H. (2015). What works for whom? Genetic moderation of intervention efficacy. *Development and Psychopathology, 27*(1), 1–6. https://doi.org/10.1017/S0954579414001254

Black, K., & Lobo, M. (2008). A conceptual review of family resilience factors. *Journal of Family Nursing, 14*(1), 33–55. https://doi.org/10.1177/1074840707312237

Bradley, R. G., Binder, E. B., Epstein, M. P., Tang, Y., Nair, H. P., Liu, W., … Ressler, K. J. (2008). Influence of child abuse on adult depression: Moderation by the corticotropin-releasing hormone receptor gene. *Archives of General Psychiatry, 65*(2), 190. https://doi.org/10.1001/archgenpsychiatry.2007.26

Brody, G. H., Beach, S. R. H., Philibert, R. A., Chen, Y., Lei, M.-K., Murry, V. M., & Brown, A. C. (2009). Parenting moderates a genetic vulnerability factor in longitudinal increases in youths' substance use. *Journal of Consulting and Clinical Psychology, 77*(1), 1–11. https://doi.org/10.1037/a0012996

Brody, G. H., Beach, S. R. H., Philibert, R. a., Chen, Y., & Murry, V. M. (2009). Prevention effects moderate the association of 5-HTTLPR and youth risk behavior initiation: Gene × environment hypotheses tested via a randomized prevention design. *Child Development, 80*(3), 645–661. https://doi.org/10.1111/j.1467-8624.2009.01288.x

Caspi, A., McClay, J., Moffitt, T. E., Mill, J., Martin, J., Craig, I. W., … Poulton, R. (2002). Role of genotype in the cycle of violence in maltreated children. *Science, 297*(5582), 851–854. https://doi.org/10.1126/science.1072290

Caspi, A., Sugden, K., Moffitt, T. E., Taylor, A., Craig, I. W., Harrington, H., … Poulton, R. (2003). Influence of life stress on depression: Moderation by a polymorphism in the 5-HTT gene. *Science, 301*(5631), 386–389. https://doi.org/10.1126/science.1083968

Chen, J., Lipska, B. K., Halim, N., Ma, Q. D., Matsumoto, M., Melhem, S., … Weinberger, D. R. (2004). Functional analysis of genetic variation in Catechol-O-Methyltransferase (COMT): Effects on mRNA, protein, and enzyme activity in postmortem human brain. *The American Journal of Human Genetics, 75*(5), 807–821. https://doi.org/10.1086/425589

Chen, L.-S., Baker, T. B., Piper, M. E., Breslau, N., Cannon, D. S., Doheny, K. F., … Bierut, L. J. (2012). Interplay of genetic risk factors (CHRNA5 - CHRNA3 - CHRNB4) and cessation treatments in smoking cessation success. *American Journal of Psychiatry, 169*(7), 735–742. https://doi.org/10.1176/appi.ajp.2012.11101545

Cicchetti, D. (2010). Resilience under conditions of extreme stress: A multilevel perspective. *World Psychiatry, 9*(3), 145–154. https://doi.org/10.1002/j.2051-5545.2010.tb00297.x

Cleveland, H. H. (2003). Disadvantaged neighborhoods and adolescent aggression: Behavioral genetic evidence of contextual effects. *Journal of Research on Adolescence, 13*(2), 211–238. https://doi.org/10.1111/1532-7795.1302004

Cleveland, H. H., Schlomer, G. L., Vandenbergh, D. J., Feinberg, M., Greenberg, M., Spoth, R., … Hair, K. L. (2015). The conditioning of intervention effects on early adolescent alcohol use by maternal involvement and dopamine receptor D4 (DRD4) and serotonin transporter linked polymorphic region (5-HTTLPR) genetic variants. *Development and Psychopathology, 27*(1), 51–67. https://doi.org/10.1017/S0954579414001291

Cleveland, H. H., Schlomer, G. L., Vandenbergh, D. J., & Wiebe, R. P. (2016). Gene × Intervention designs: A promising step toward understanding eitiology and building better preventive interventions. *Criminology and Public Policy, 15*(3), 711–720. https://doi.org/10.1111/1745-9133.12221

Cleveland, H. H., Griffin, A. M., Wolf, P. S. A., Wiebe, R. P., Schlomer, G. L., Feinberg, M. E., … Vandenbergh, D. J. (2018). Transactions between substance use intervention, the oxytocin receptor (OXTR) gene, and peer substance use predicting youth alcohol use. *Prevention Science, 19*(1), 15–26. https://doi.org/10.1007/s11121-017-0749-5

Cleveland, H. H., Schlomer, G. L., Vandenbergh, D. J., Wolf, P. S. A., Feinberg, M. E., Greenberg, M. T., … Redmond, C. (2018). Associations between alcohol dehydrogenase genes and alcohol use across early and middle adolescence: Moderation × Preventive intervention. *Development and Psychopathology, 30*(1), 297–313. https://doi.org/10.1017/S0954579417000633

Cleveland, H. H., & Wiebe, R. P. (2003). The moderation of genetic and shared-environmental influences on adolescent drinking by levels of parental drinking. *Journal of Studies on Alcohol, 64*(2), 182–194.

Collins, L. M., Murphy, S. A., & Strecher, V. (2007). The multiphase optimization strategy (MOST) and the sequential multiple assignment randomized trial (SMART). *American Journal of Preventive Medicine, 32*(5), S112–S118. https://doi.org/10.1016/j.amepre.2007.01.022

Creswell, K. G., Sayette, M. A., Manuck, S. B., Ferrell, R. E., Hill, S. Y., & Dimoff, J. D. (2012). DRD4 polymorphism moderates the effect of alcohol consumption on social bonding. *PLoS One, 7*(2), e28914. https://doi.org/10.1371/journal.pone.0028914

Crick, F. H. (1958). On protein synthesis. *Symposia of the Society for Experimental Biology, 12*, 138–163. https://doi.org/10.1038/227561a0

Culverhouse, R. C., Saccone, N. L., Horton, A. C., Ma, Y., Anstey, K. J., Banaschewski, T., … Bierut, L. J. (2017). Collaborative meta-analysis finds no evidence of a strong interaction between stress and 5-HTTLPR genotype contributing to the development of depression. *Molecular Psychiatry*, 1–10. https://doi.org/10.1038/mp.2017.44

Daw, N. D., Kakade, S., & Dayan, P. (2002). Opponent interactions between serotonin and dopamine. *Neural Networks, 15*, 603–616. https://doi.org/10.1016/S0893-6080(02)00052-7

Dick, D. M., Agrawal, A., Keller, M. C., Adkins, A., Aliev, F., Monroe, S., … Sher, K. J. (2015). Candidate gene-environment interaction research: Reflections and recommendations. *Perspectives on Psychological Science, 10*(1), 37–59. https://doi.org/10.1177/1745691614556682

Duncan, L. E., & Keller, M. C. (2011). A critical review of the first 10 years of candidate gene-by-environment interaction research in psychiatry. *American Journal of Psychiatry, 168*(10), 1041–1049. https://doi.org/10.1176/appi.ajp.2011.11020191

Edenberg, H. J., & Foroud, T. (2014). Genetics of alcoholism. In *Handbook of clinical neurology* (Vol. 125, pp. 561–571). Waltham, MA: Elsevier. https://doi.org/10.1016/B978-0-444-62619-6.00032-X

Egeland, B., Carlson, E., & Sroufe, L. A. (1993). Resilience as process. *Development and Psychopathology, 5*(4), 517–528. https://doi.org/10.1017/S0954579400006131

Elam, K. K., Wang, F., Bountress, K., Chassin, L., Lemery-Chalfant, K., Dick, D., ... Sher, K. (2014, November). Using a literature-based polygenic risk score for behavioral undercontrol to examine evocative genotypeenvironment correlation. In *Behavior Genetics* (Vol. 44, No. 6, pp. 657–657). New York, NY: Springer.

Elam, K. I. T. K., Wang, F. L., Bountress, K., Chassin, L., Pandika, D., & Lemery-chalfant, K. (2016). Predicting substance use in emerging adulthood: A genetically informed study of developmental transactions between impulsivity and family conflict. *Development and Psychopathology, 28*, 673–688. https://doi.org/10.1017/S0954579416000249

Elam, K. K., Chassin, L., Lemery-Chalfant, K., Pandika, D., Wang, F. L., Bountress, K., ... & Agrawal, A. (2017). Affiliation with substance-using peers: Examining gene-environment correlations among parent monitoring, polygenic risk, and children's impulsivity. *Developmental psychobiology, 59*(5), 561–573.

Ellis, B. J., Boyce, W. T., Belsky, J., Bakermans-Kranenburg, M. J., & van Ijzendoorn, M. H. (2011). Differential susceptibility to the environment: An evolutionary–neurodevelopmental theory. *Development and Psychopathology, 23*(1), 7–28. https://doi.org/10.1017/S0954579410000611

Fosco, G. M., DeBoard, R. L., & Grych, J. H. (2007). Making sense of family violence: Implications of children's appraisals of interparental aggression for their short- and long-term functioning. *European Psychologist, 12*(1), 6–16. https://doi.org/10.1027/1016-9040.12.1.6

Freedman, M. L., Reich, D., Penney, K. L., McDonald, G. J., Mignault, A. A., Patterson, N., … Altshuler, D. (2004). Assessing the impact of population stratification on genetic association studies. *Nature Genetics, 36*(4), 388–393. https://doi.org/10.1038/ng1333

Fullerton, S. M., Yu, J. H., Crouch, J., Fryer-Edwards, K., & Burke, W. (2010). Population description and its role in the interpretation of genetic association. *Human Genetics, 127*(5), 563–572. https://doi.org/10.1007/s00439-010-0800-0

Gajos, J. M., Fagan, A. A., & Beaver, K. M. (2016). Use of genetically informed evidence-based prevention science to understand and prevent crime and related behavioral disorders. *Criminology & Public Policy, 15*(3), 683–701. https://doi.org/10.1111/1745-9133.12214

Halder, I., Shriver, M., Thomas, M., Fernandez, J. R., & Frudakis, T. (2008). A panel of ancestry informative markers for estimating individual biogeographical ancestry and admixture from four continents: Utility and applications. *Human Mutation, 29*(5), 648–658. https://doi.org/10.1002/humu.20695

Howe, G. W., Beach, S. R. H., & Brody, G. H. (2010). Microtrial methods for translating gene-environment dynamics into preventive interventions. *Prevention Science, 11*(4), 343–354. https://doi.org/10.1007/s11121-010-0177-2

Iacono, W. G., Malone, S. M., & McGue, M. (2008). Behavioral disinhibition and the development of early-onset addiction: Common and specific Influences. *Annual Review of Clinical Psychology, 4*(1), 325–348. https://doi.org/10.1146/annurev.clinpsy.4.022007.141157

Janssens, A., Van Den Noortgate, W., Goossens, L., Verschueren, K., Colpin, H., De Laet, S., … Van Leeuwen, K. (2015). Externalizing problem behavior in adolescence: Dopaminergic genes in interaction with peer acceptance and rejection. *Journal of Youth and Adolescence, 44*(7), 1441–1456. https://doi.org/10.1007/s10964-015-0304-2

Kapur, S., & Remington, G. (1996). Serotonin-dopamine interactions and Its relevance to schizophrenia. *American Journal of Psychiatry, 153*(4), 466–476. https://doi.org/10.1176/ajp.153.4.466

Karg, K., Burmeister, M., Shedden, K., & Sen, S. (2011). The serotonin transporter promoter variant (5-HTTLPR), stress, and depression meta-analysis revisited: Evidence of genetic moderation. *Archives of General Psychiatry, 68*(5), 444–454. https://doi.org/10.1001/archgenpsychiatry.2010.189

Knerr, S., Wayman, D., & Bonham, V. L. (2011). Inclusion of racial and ethnic minorities in genetic research: Advance the spirit by changing the rules? *Journal of Law, Medicine and Ethics, 39*(3), 502–512. https://doi.org/10.1111/j.1748-720X.2011.00617.x

Larsen, H., van der Zwaluw, C. S., Overbeek, G., Granic, I., Franke, B., & Engels, R. C. M. E. (2010). A variable-number-of-tandem-repeats polymorphism in the dopamine D4 receptor gene affects social adaptation of alcohol use: Investigation of a gene-environment interaction. *Psychological Science, 21*(8), 1064–1068. https://doi.org/10.1177/0956797610376654

Leve, L. D., Harold, G. T., Ge, X., Neiderhiser, J. M., & Patterson, G. (2010). Refining intervention targets in family-based research: Lessons from quantitative behavioral genetics. *Perspectives on Psychological Science, 5*(5), 516–526. https://doi.org/10.1177/1745691610383506

Luan, J. a., Wong, M. Y., Day, N. E., & Wareham, N. J. (2001). Sample size determination for studies of gene-environment interaction. *International Journal of Epidemiology, 30*(5), 1035–1040. https://doi.org/10.1093/ije/30.5.1035

Luthar, S. S., Cicchetti, D., & Becker, B. (2000). The construct of resilience: A critical evaluation and guidelines for future work. *Child Development, 71*(3), 543–562. https://doi.org/10.1111/1467-8624.00164

Luthar, S. S., & Zigler, E. (1991). Vulnerability and competence: A review of research on resilience in childhood. *The American Journal of Orthopsychiatry, 61*(1), 6–22. https://doi.org/10.1037/h0079218

Malik, A. I., Zai, C. C., Abu, Z., Nowrouzi, B., & Beitchman, J. H. (2012). The role of oxytocin and oxytocin receptor gene variants in childhood-onset aggression. *Genes, brain and behavior, 11*(5), 545–551

Mannucci, A., Sullivan, K. M., Ivanov, P. L., & Gill, P. (1994). Forensic application of a rapid and quantitative DNA sex test by amplification of the X-Y homologous gene amelogenin. *International Journal of Legal Medicine, 106*(4), 190–193. https://doi.org/10.1007/BF01371335

Manolio, T. A., Collins, F. S., Cox, N. J., Goldstein, D. B., Hindorff, L. A., Hunter, D. J., … Visscher, P. M. (2009). Finding the missing heritability of complex diseases. *Nature, 461*(7265), 747–753. https://doi.org/10.1038/nature08494

Manuck, S. B., & McCaffery, J. M. (2014). Gene-environment interaction. *Annual Review of Psychology, 65*(1), 41–70. https://doi.org/10.1146/annurev-psych-010213-115100
Masten, A., Hubbard, J. J., Gest, S. D., Tellegen, A., Garmezy, N., & Ramirez, M. (1999). Competence in the context of adversity: Pathways to resilience and maladaptation from childhood to late adolescence. *Development and Psychopathology, 11*(1), 143–169. https://doi.org/10.1017/S0954579499001996
Masten, A. S. (2001). Ordinary magic: Resilience processes in development. *American Psychologist, 56*(3), 227–238. https://doi.org/10.1037//0003-066X.56.3.227
Masten, A. S., Best, K. M., & Garmezy, N. (1990). Resilience and development: Contributions from the study of children who overcome adversity. *Development and Psychopathology, 2*(4), 425–444. https://doi.org/10.1017/S0954579400005812
Masten, A. S., & Obradović, J. (2006). Competence and resilience in development. *Annals of the New York Academy of Sciences, 1094*(1), 13–27. https://doi.org/10.1196/annals.1376.003
Maurano, M. T., Humbert, R., Rynes, E., Thurman, R. E., Haugen, E., Wang, H., … Stamatoyannopoulos, J. A. (2012). Systematic localization of common disease-associated variation in regulatory DNA. *Science, 337*(6099), 1190–1195. https://doi.org/10.1126/science.1222794
McClelland, G. H., & Judd, C. M. (1993). Statistical difficulties of detecting interactions and moderator effects. *Psychological Bulletin, 114*(2), 376–390. https://doi.org/10.1037/0033-2909.114.2.376
Monroe, S., & Simons, A. (1991). Diathesis-stress theories in the context of life stress research: Implications for the depressive disorders. *Psychological Bulletin, 110*(3), 406–425.
Monroe, S. M., & Reid, M. (2008). Gene-environment interactions in depression research genetic polymorphisms and life-stress polyprocedures. *Psychological Science, 19*(10), 947–957. https://doi.org/10.1111/j.1467-9280.2008.02181.x
Munafò, M. R. (2006). Candidate gene studies in the 21st century: Meta-analysis, mediation, moderation. *Genes, Brain, and Behavior, 5*(Suppl 1), 3–8. https://doi.org/10.1111/j.1601-183X.2006.00188.x
Munafò, M. R., Durrant, C., Lewis, G., & Flint, J. (2009). Gene × environment interactions at the serotonin transporter locus. *Biological Psychiatry, 65*(3), 211–219. https://doi.org/10.1016/j.biopsych.2008.06.009
Musci, R. J., Masyn, K. E., Uhl, G., Maher, B., Kellam, S. G., & Ialongo, N. S. (2015). Polygenic score x intervention moderation: An application of discrete-time survival analysis to modeling the timing of first tobacco use among urban youth. *Development and Psychopathology, 27*(1), 111–122. https://doi.org/10.1038/leu.2015.15\r10.1017/s0954579414001333
Musci, R. J., & Schlomer, G. L. (2017). The implications of genetics for prevention and intervention programming. *Prevention Science, 19*, 1–5. https://doi.org/10.1007/s11121-017-0837-6
Nicolae, D. L., Gamazon, E., Zhang, W., Duan, S., Eileen Dolan, M., & Cox, N. J. (2010). Trait-associated SNPs are more likely to be eQTLs: Annotation to enhance discovery from GWAS. *PLoS Genetics, 6*(4), e1000888. https://doi.org/10.1371/journal.pgen.1000888
Nikolova, Y. S., Ferrell, R. E., Manuck, S. B., & Hariri, A. R. (2011). Multilocus genetic profile for dopamine signaling predicts ventral striatum reactivity. *Neuropsychopharmacology, 36*(9), 1940–1947. https://doi.org/10.1038/npp.2011.82
Perkel, J. (2008). SNP genotyping: Six technologies that keyed a revolution. *Nature Methods, 5*(5), 575–575. https://doi.org/10.1038/nmeth0608-575b
Preacher, K. J., Curran, P. J., & Bauer, D. J. (2006). Computational tools for probing interactions in multiple linear regression, multilevel modeling, and latent curve analysis. *Journal of Educational and Behavioral Statistics, 31*(4), 437–448. https://doi.org/10.3102/10769986031004437
Purcell, S., Neale, B., Todd-Brown, K., Thomas, L., Ferreira, M. A. R., Bender, D., … Sham, P. C. (2007). PLINK: A tool set for whole-genome association and population-based linkage analyses. *The American Journal of Human Genetics, 81*(3), 559–575. https://doi.org/10.1086/519795
Reiss, D., & Leve, L. D. (2007). Genetic expression outside the skin: Clues to mechanisms of genotype × environment interaction. *Development and Psychopathology, 19*(4), 181–204. https://doi.org/10.1017/S0954579407000508

Reiss, D., Leve, L. D., & Neiderhiser, J. M. (2013). How genes and the social environment moderate each other. *American Journal of Public Health, 103*(Suppl.1), 1–10. https://doi.org/10.2105/AJPH.2013.301408

Risch, N., Herrell, R., Lehner, T., Liang, K. Y., Eaves, L., Hoh, J., … Merikangas, K. R. (2009). Interaction between the serotonin transporter gene (5-HTTLPR), stressful life events, and risk of depression: A meta-analysis. *Jama, 301*(23), 2462–2472. https://doi.org/10.1001/jama.2009.878

Roisman, G. I., Newman, D. A., Fraley, R. C., Haltigan, J. D., Groh, A. M., & Haydon, K. C. (2012). Distinguishing differential susceptibility from diathesis–stress: Recommendations for evaluating interaction effects. *Development and Psychopathology, 24*(2), 389–409. https://doi.org/10.1017/S0954579412000065

Russell, M. A., Schlomer, G. L., Cleveland, H. H., Feinberg, M. E., Greenberg, M. T., Spoth, R. L., … Vandenbergh, D. J. (2018). PROSPER intervention effects on adolescents' alcohol misuse vary by GABRA2 genotype and age. *Prevention Science, 19*(1), 27–37. https://doi.org/10.1007/s11121-017-0751-y

Rutter, M. (1987). Psychosocial resilience and protective mechanisms. *American Journal of Orthopsychiatry, 57*(3), 316–331. https://doi.org/10.1111/j.1939-0025.1987.tb03541.x

Rutter, M. (1993). Resilience: Some conceptual considerations. *Journal of Adolescent Health, 14*(8), 626–631. https://doi.org/10.1016/1054-139X(93)90196-V

Rutter, M. (2012). Resilience as a dynamic concept. *Development and Psychopathology, 24*, 335–344. https://doi.org/10.1017/S0954579412000028

Rutter, M., Thapar, A., & Pickles, A. (2009). Gene-environment interactions. *Archives of General Psychiatry, 66*(12), 1287–1289. https://doi.org/10.1001/archgenpsychiatry.2009.167

Salvatore, J. E., & Dick, D. M. (2015). Gene-environment interplay: Where we are, where we are going. *Journal of Marriage and Family, 77*(2), 344–350. https://doi.org/10.1111/jomf.12164

Scarr, S., & McCartney, K. (1983). How people make their own environments: A theory of genotype environment effects. *Child Development, 54*(2), 424–435. https://doi.org/10.2307/1129703

Schlomer, G. L., Cleveland, H. H., Feinberg, M. E., Wolf, P. S., Greenberg, M. T., Spoth, R. L., ... & Vandenbergh, D. J. (2017). Extending previous cG× I findings on 5-HTTLPR's moderation of intervention effects on adolescent substance misuse initiation. *Child Development, 88*(6), 2001–2012. https://doi.org/10.1111/cdev.12666

Schlomer, G. L., Cleveland, H. H., Vandenbergh, D. J., Fosco, G. M., & Feinberg, M. E. (2015). Looking forward in candidate gene research: Concerns and suggestions. *Journal of Marriage and Family, 77*(2), 351–354. https://doi.org/10.1111/jomf.12165

Schlomer, G. L., Cleveland, H. H., Vandenbergh, D. J., Wolf, P. S. A., Feinberg, M. E., & Greenberg, M. T. (n.d.). 5-HTTLPR moderates intervention effects on early adolescent substance abuse initiation. *Child Development.*

Schlomer, G. L., Fosco, G. M., Cleveland, H. H., Vandenbergh, D. J., & Feinberg, M. E. (2015). Interparental relationship sensitivity leads to adolescent internalizing problems: Different genotypes, different pathways. *Journal of Marriage and Family, 77*(2), 329–343. https://doi.org/10.1111/jomf.12168

Schoots, O., & Van Tol, H. H. M. (2003). The human dopamine D4 receptor repeat sequences modulate expression. *The Pharmacogenomics Journal, 3*(6), 343–348. https://doi.org/10.1038/sj.tpj.6500208

Stephens, S. H., Hartz, S. M., Hoft, N. R., Saccone, N. L., Corley, R. C., Hewitt, J. K., … Ehringer, M. A. (2013). Distinct loci in the CHRNA5/CHRNA3/CHRNB4 gene cluster are associated with onset of regular smoking. *Genetic Epidemiology, 37*(8), 846–859. https://doi.org/10.1002/gepi.21760

Turkheimer, E. (2000). Three laws of behavior genetics and what they mean. *Current Directions in Psychological Science, 9*(5), 160–164. https://doi.org/10.1111/1467-8721.00084

Uher, R., & McGuffin, P. (2008). The moderation by the serotonin transporter gene of environmental adversity in the aetiology of mental illness: Review and methodological analysis. *Molecular Psychiatry, 13*(2), 131–146. https://doi.org/10.1038/sj.mp.4002067

Uher, R., & McGuffin, P. (2010). The moderation by the serotonin transporter gene of environmental adversity in the etiology of depression: 2009 update. *Molecular Psychiatry, 15*(1), 18–22. https://doi.org/10.1038/mp.2009.123

Uhl, G. R., Drgon, T., Johnson, C., Ramoni, M. F., Behm, F. M., & Rose, J. E. (2010). Genome-wide association for smoking cessation success in a trial of precessation nicotine replacement. *Molecular Medicine, 16*(11), 513–526. https://doi.org/10.2119/molmed.2010.00052

Uhl, G. R., Walther, D., Musci, R., Fisher, C., Anthony, J. C., Storr, C. L., … Rose, J. E. (2014). Smoking quit success genotype score predicts quit success and distinct patterns of developmental involvement with common addictive substances. *Molecular Psychiatry, 19*(1), 50–54. https://doi.org/10.1038/mp.2012.155

Van Ijzendoorn, M. H., Bakermans-Kranenburg, M. J., Belsky, J., Beach, S., Brody, G., Dodge, K. A., … Scott, S. (2011). Gene-by-environment experiments: A new approach to finding the missing heritability. *Nature Reviews Genetics, 12*(12), 881–881. https://doi.org/10.1038/nrg2764-c1

Vandenbergh, D. J., & Schlomer, G. L. (2014). Finding genomic function for genetic associations in nicotine addiction research: The ENCODE project's role in future pharmacogenomic analysis. *Pharmacology Biochemistry and Behavior, 123*(5), 34–44. https://doi.org/10.1016/j.pbb.2014.01.009

Vandenbergh, D. J., Schlomer, G. L., Cleveland, H. H., Schink, A. E., Hair, K. L., Feinberg, M. E., … & Redmond, C. (2015). An adolescent substance prevention model blocks the effect of CHRNA5 genotype on smoking during high school. *Nicotine & Tobacco Research, 18*(2), 212–220.

Villafuerte, S., Trucco, E. M., Heitzeg, M. M., Burmeister, M., & Zucker, R. A. (2014). Genetic variation in GABRA2 moderates peer influence on externalizing behavior in adolescents. *Brain and Behavior, 4*(6), 833–840. https://doi.org/10.1002/brb3.291

Wang, T., & Elston, R. C. (2005). Two-level Haseman-Elston regression for general pedigree data analysis. *Genetic Epidemiology, 29*(1), 12–22. https://doi.org/10.1002/gepi.20075

Widaman, K. F., Helm, J. L., Castro-Schilo, L., Pluess, M., Stallings, M. C., & Belsky, J. (2012). Distinguishing ordinal and disordinal interactions. *Psychological Methods, 17*(4), 615–622. https://doi.org/10.1037/a0030003

Wong, P. T.-H., Feng, H., & Teo, W. L. (1995). Interaction of the dopaminergic and serotonergic systems in the rat striatum: Effects of selective antagonists and uptake inhibitors. *Neuroscience Research, 23*(1), 115–119. https://doi.org/10.1016/0168-0102(95)90023-3

Yacubian, J., Sommer, T., Schroeder, K., Gläscher, J., Kalisch, R., Leuenberger, B., … Büchel, C. (2007). Gene-gene interaction associated with neural reward sensitivity. *Proceedings of the National Academy of Sciences of the United States of America, 104*(19), 8125–8130. https://doi.org/10.1073/pnas.0702029104

Zakhari, S. (2006). Overview: How is alcohol metabolized by the body? *Alcohol Research & Health, 29*(4), 245–254.

Chapter 8
Risk as a First Derivative: Using Intensive Repeated Measures and Molecular Approaches to Studying Families

Theodore F. Robles

> *In calculus, the first derivative of a point is not its position in space, but its propensity to change its position; not where an object is, but how it moves in space and time*
>
> *Mukherjee (2015, p. 355).*

The ups and downs of family life act through biobehavioral mechanisms to influence physical health (Miller & Chen, 2010; Repetti, Robles, & Reynolds, 2011). This chapter describes how multiple repeated measures of those "ups and downs," when combined with measures of biologically plausible mechanisms like the hypothalamic-pituitary-adrenal axis and immune system function (Miller, Chen, & Cole, 2009), can yield insights into how individuals respond to challenges in the family and in the body, which can ultimately inform understanding of risk and resilience.

The quote that opened this chapter refers to a "first derivative" in mathematics, which is the instantaneous slope of a function, reflecting the change in *Y* per unit of *X*. This is illustrated in Fig. 8.1 with a scatterplot of hypothetical data, with variable *X* on the *x*-axis and variable *Y* on the *y*-axis, and a best-fit line running through the points. In calculus, the first derivative test can determine whether a critical point is a minimum, maximum, or neither; in physics, the derivative of the position of a moving object with respect to time is its velocity; in the current chapter's conceptualization, a function representing how parent–child conflict is related to other variables and how it changes over time is assessed. With intensive repeated measures of parent–child conflict as the *Y*, over *X* repeated days, researchers can differentiate change in parent–child conflict between family units, often described as slopes of change over time. This traditional way of thinking about intensive repeated measures

T. F. Robles (✉)
Department of Psychology, University of California, Los Angeles, Los Angeles, CA, USA
e-mail: robles@psych.ucla.edu

A. W. Harrist, B. C. Gardner (eds.), *Biobehavioral Markers in Risk and Resilience Research*, Emerging Issues in Family and Individual Resilience,
https://doi.org/10.1007/978-3-030-05952-1_8

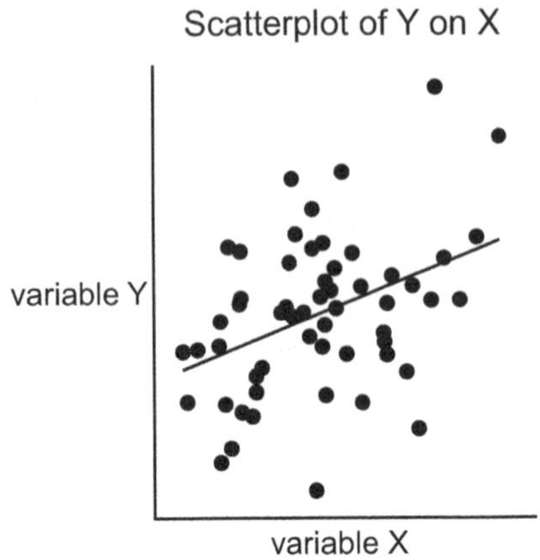

Fig. 8.1 Scatterplot of two variables (*X* and *Y*), where the slope of the best-fit line through the points represents a "first derivative"

can be extended to measuring two variables over time, such as negative mood as the *Y*, and parent–child conflict as *X*; importantly, each point on the scatterplot in Fig. 8.1 would then represent a given day in the study. The best-fit line then represents the person-level correlation between *X* and *Y* during a particular time period, which I describe as within-person associations. In these examples, both types of derivatives, change over time, and within-person associations can be viewed as "potential" for change over time or over within-person changes in parent–child conflict. In addition to using intensive repeated psychosocial measures to evaluate "potential" to respond, this paper also describes ways to possibly infer how the immune system might respond to threats, something that may be important for understanding links between health and family functioning in the future. Thus, the purpose of this chapter is to highlight the benefit of using intensive repeated measures approaches to studying families to conceptualize risk for poor health. Rather than providing "snapshots" of family functioning, maximizing the use of intensive repeated measures may provide more precise yet efficient estimates of risk and resilience in families. The chapter also describes the value of genomic approaches to illuminate common immune pathways that may be markers of risk or resilience.

8.1 Foundational Points Regarding Research Design

Much of this volume focuses on biological measures as outcomes and potential risk/resilience markers. Incorporation of biological measures in behavioral research should address known biological processes of disease risk *and* the relevance of the objective biological measurement to the outcome of interest. Some biological measures represent surrogate endpoints that based on empirical evidence can substitute for clinical endpoints, which often require the passage of time, making the use of surrogate endpoints more temporally appropriate, based on current understanding of biological processes of disease (Biomarker Definitions Working Group, 2001).

For instance, across numerous studies, levels of LDL or the so-called bad cholesterol predict cardiovascular disease onset as well as progression of disease, including cardiac events like having a second heart attack (Vasan, 2006). Thus, many clinical trials have examined LDL cholesterol as a primary outcome, rather than following participants through the development of disease. Plausible biological processes also suggest other biomarkers of psychosocial factors that influence health, but are not specifically diagnostic or prognostic for specific health outcomes. Many of those *biological mediators* that reflect allostatic processes (responses to environmental demands) may be common across health conditions (Robles & Carroll, 2011), and the vast majority of biomarkers described in this volume and all the markers in this chapter refer to biological mediators.

Biomarkers that reflect allostatic processes are often described as potential measures of stress exposure (Harkness & Monroe, 2016), or resilience to such exposure. However, allostatic processes like the hypothalamic-pituitary-adrenal axis and immune function respond to a variety of stimuli, ranging from stressful life events to infections. Accordingly, inferring stress exposures from biological responses, or more specifically, exposures to conflict or support in the family environment from biological responses, is not sound practice (Cacioppo & Tassinary, 1990; Harkness & Monroe, 2016). Put another way, if low levels of inflammation are viewed as resilience to stressful circumstances, that inference cannot be made without knowing whether such individuals were actually exposed to such circumstances. The ability to infer "psychological significance from physiological signals" (Cacioppo & Tassinary, 1990) is an aspirational goal, but peripheral biological markers that reflect allostatic processes are the output of multiple layers of processing at multiple levels of the brain (Ulrich-Lai & Herman, 2009), and because of that, simply knowing that an individual has an average of 3.19 μg/dL of cortisol in the evening cannot tell us about the type, duration, or course of stressful life events and circumstances the person is exposed to. Accordingly, both stress exposures and allostatic processes must be measured in the same study (Harkness & Monroe, 2016). In the context of family environments, understanding both stressful and supportive aspects of the family become critical for inferring how families impact health through direct biological influences.

Everyday family circumstances are primarily assessed using self-report, in part because of the difficulty inherent in conducting systematic behavioral observations in the home (Repetti, Reynolds, & Sears, 2015). However, objective systematic observations of family experiences can be captured through Electronically Activated Recorder (Slatcher & Robles, 2012), and in-person observations (reviewed in Repetti et al., 2015). This paper focuses on self-report measures because of their ease of use relative to objective methods, as well as their value in assessing social-cognitive and affective responses to events in the home. Using intensive repeated measures of the family environment, relative to single, retrospective, and infrequently administered self-report measures (i.e., "how often in the last month did you argue with your spouse?") offers several advantages: reduced recall and retrospection bias, increased relevance for interventions, and greater ability to use sophisticated quantitative approaches (see Repetti et al., 2015 for a comprehensive review).

To illustrate these advantages, I describe two applications of intensive repeated measures from the UCLA Families and Health study, a prospective daily diary study of 47 families with children between 8 and 13 years of age (Robles, Reynolds, Repetti, & Chung, 2013). Both applications involve moving beyond static snapshots of exposure to "first derivative" conceptualizations of how family environments change over time, and how children respond to such changes.

8.2 UCLA Families and Health Study Participants and Procedures

Briefly, families with children 8–13 years old were recruited in the Los Angeles area from 2009 to 2012 to participate in a study during the fall and winter months, which corresponds to the cold and flu season in Los Angeles county (Robles et al., 2018). Children had to be free of medical conditions that could confound endocrine and immune measures, including chronic lung conditions, endocrine and metabolic disorders, immunodeficiency, and cardiovascular disease. Of 60 families that were eligible to participate, 47 were enrolled in the study, and include 47 mothers, 39 fathers, 47 target children (28 female), and 12 siblings (7 female) who were in the target age range (for more details, see Robles et al., 2018). Families were majority-minority (55% of parents were people of color), average parent age was mid-40s, just over 50% of the sample had a 4-year college degree or higher, and 80% of fathers and 45% of mothers worked full-time.

A timeline of the study procedures is shown in Fig. 8.2. Participating parents and target children completed the UCLA Life Stress Interview, which assesses stressful life events and circumstances, as well as questionnaire measures of the family environment during a home visit. During a subsequent visit, parents and children were trained on how to complete online daily diary questionnaires and provide saliva samples. The following Saturday, participants completed the 8-week daily diary portion of the study (More details regarding compliance and measurement issues can be found in Reynolds, Robles, & Repetti, 2016). During weeks 3 and 6, four saliva samples were collected on four consecutive days (Saturday–Tuesday) for salivary cortisol assays (Kuhlman, Repetti, Reynolds, & Robles, 2016). At the end of the study, parents and children that opted to provide a blood sample did so, and children completed a brief laboratory stressor in our laboratory.

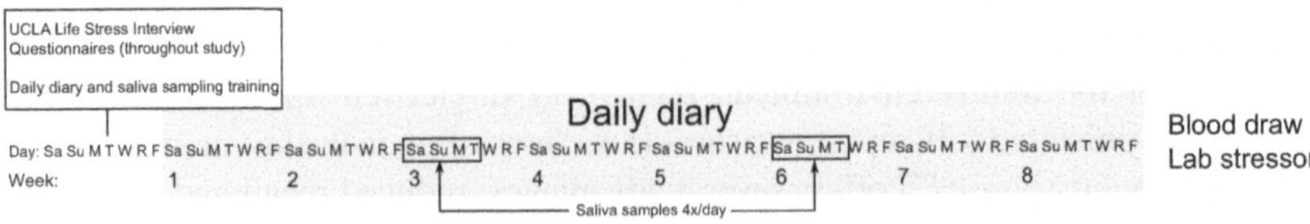

Fig. 8.2 Timeline of procedures in the UCLA Families and Health Study

8.2.1 "First Derivative" Approaches to Characterizing Exposures

8.2.1.1 Change in Family Functioning Over Time and HPA Axis Function

The unique saliva sampling protocol in the study allowed for examining how changes in the family environment may be related to changes in HPA axis function and regulation over short timeframes (e.g., weeks). Identifying the timeframe over which family environments and changes in those environments are related to HPA axis function has direct implications for psychosocial interventions that examine HPA axis measures as outcomes (Slopen, McLaughlin, & Shonkoff, 2014). For instance, if the HPA axis is insensitive to week-to-week or month-to-month changes in the family environment, such as improving parent–child relationships during a family intervention, then pre- to post-measures of cortisol may not be an appropriate outcome; more long-term post-intervention follow-up may be needed to observe biologically plausible and relevant changes.

On the other hand, if the HPA axis is sensitive to short-term fluctuations in the family environment, measuring cortisol changes over shorter intervals, like pre- to post-intervention, may provide a relevant window for understanding the role of biological processes in mediating intervention effects. The existing literature to date has examined day-to-day changes in cortisol as a function of family environments over a week or so (e.g., Lippold, McHale, Davis, Almeida, & King, 2016), but not over longer timeframes. Accordingly, our study design allowed examination of changes in HPA axis regulation from Week 3 to Week 6, as a function of changes in child-reported parent–child conflict from Week 1 to Week 2, and from Week 4 to Week 6. We hypothesized that increasing parent–child conflict over time would be related to upregulated HPA axis activity, reflected in larger cortisol awakening responses, higher daily cortisol output (area under the curve ground, AUCg), flatter diurnal cortisol slopes, and higher bedtime cortisol (Kuhlman et al., 2016).

Daily parent–child conflict was assessed by asking children six items from the Youth Everyday Social Interaction and Mood scales (Lehman & Repetti, 2007; Repetti, 1996), including "My mom/dad got mad at me today," "My mom/dad punished me today," and "I was angry at mom/dad today." Week 1 to Week 2 change was characterized by computing individual slopes of change in parent–child conflict reports from day 1 to 16, and Week 4 to 6 change was characterized by computing slopes of change from day 22 to 37 (Kuhlman et al., 2016). Notably, conflict was an occasional event, reported on 33% of study days. On average, conflict levels decreased over the course of the study from 1.20 ($SD = 0.31$) on a 1 (not at all) to 3 (a lot) scale after averaging across the six items, by a rate of −0.005 units per day. While conflict was occasional, 48% of children showed an increase in parent–child conflict from Week 1 to Week 2, and 60% showed an increase from Week 4 to Week 6.

The primary finding was that increased parent–child conflict from Week 4 to Week 6 was related to increases in daily cortisol output and a flattened diurnal cortisol slope from Week 3 to Week 6, all of which were likely accounted for by increases in bedtime cortisol. Children who showed a 1 *SD* increase in parent–child conflict showed an increase in bedtime cortisol from Week 3 to Week 6, whereas children who showed a decrease in parent–child conflict showed no change in bedtime cortisol. In additional analyses, we found that longer periods of daily diary sampling (16 days vs. 14, 9, or 3 days) were needed to observe associations between change in parent–child conflict and daily cortisol output and bedtime cortisol, whereas shorter periods of sampling (particular 3 days) were needed to observe associations between changes in parent–child conflict and diurnal cortisol slope. Overall, these findings suggested that certain parameters of HPA axis function (daily output and bedtime cortisol) were sensitive to changes in the family environment over several weeks. Our findings also imply that changes in bedtime cortisol levels, when the HPA axis is expected to be the least "active," may be the most responsive to variations in the family environment, including variations that may be introduced through family-based interventions. The intensive repeated measures of parent–child conflict, combined with the unique two-stage sampling of cortisol on Weeks 3 and 6 allowed for testing such questions.

8.2.1.2 Using Intensive Repeated Measures to Model Mood "Reactivity" to Marital and Parent–Child Conflict and Warmth and Leukocyte Telomere Length

Intensive repeated measures provide multiple occasions of measurement over time, and when *multiple measures* over multiple occasions are obtained, can provide additional "first derivative" insights into how children respond or react to their environments. Such an approach was initially pioneered by research on adults from the National Study of Daily Experiences, in which stressful event exposures were assessed daily for 8 days, along with daily measures of negative mood. The study team computed the difference in negative mood between the day with the fewest exposures and the day with the most exposures, and used that difference as an index of participants' "emotional reactivity" to daily stressful events (e.g., Charles, Piazza, Mogle, Sliwinski, & Almeida, 2013). With 56 days in the Families and Health study, we were able to compute correlations between exposures (conflict and warmth in the family) and negative mood within each child over 2 months of sampling. Put another way, we could compute slopes of the association between exposures and negative mood for individual children in our study.

Emotional reactivity to the family environment, particularly interparental conflict, is implicated as a key mechanism linking stressful family environments to children's emotional and physical well-being (Repetti et al., 2011; Troxel & Matthews, 2004). Emotional security theory posits that children's repeated exposure to interparental conflict over time contributes to emotional insecurity, and subsequent difficulties with regulating emotions that manifest in greater affective reactivity, behavior problems (i.e., externalizing symptoms), and social-cognitive dysregulation such as persistent distrust of others (Davies & Cummings, 1994; Davies & Martin, 2013).

Greater emotional reactivity is then implicated as a contributor to risky health behaviors (e.g., substance use), dysregulated allostatic processes, with eventual deleterious effects on health and well-being (Troxel & Matthews, 2004).

Using data from the Families and Health study, we examined links between emotional reactivity to the family environment and a potential indicator of dysregulated allostatic processes: accelerated immune cell aging (Robles et al., 2016). Conceptually, cells of the immune system have a finite capacity to divide (e.g., 50–70 cell divisions), and markers of immune cell aging provide a window into how impacted immune cells are by infectious threats, normal cellular damage, and perhaps even exposure to stressful events (Puterman & Epel, 2012). Moreover, "older" immune cells may actually contribute to poorer health by promoting elevated inflammation (Campisi & di Fagagna, 2007). One marker of immune cell aging that has gained significant interest over the past two decades is telomere length; telomeres are nucleotide structures that cap the ends of chromosomes in a manner analogous to how plastic sheaths (aglets) on the end of shoelaces prevent shoelaces from fraying (Blackburn, 2000). Normal cell division results in the loss of genetic material at the end of chromosomes, and the genetic material in telomeres is sacrificed to prevent loss of genetic material that we need for survival. While telomeres can be lengthened or shortened, the general view is that shorter telomeres indicate older cells.

Emotional reactivity is more broadly implicated in models linking psychological stress to premature cellular aging, and shorter immune cell telomere length in older adults is associated with poorer health outcomes (Puterman & Epel, 2012). Such observations have led developmental researchers to explore whether stressful life event exposures are systematically related to cellular aging in children (Shalev, 2012). In several studies examining telomere length in cells that line the inside of the cheek (buccal cells), exposure to major life events involving loss, as well as longitudinal changes in parent-reported exposure to violence from ages 5 to 15 were related to shorter buccal cell telomere length (Drury et al., 2014; Shalev et al., 2013). Both aforementioned studies examined cumulative exposure to major life events, and the Families and Health data provided an opportunity to extend this line of inquiry to mild-to-moderate daily family stress exposures, emotional reactivity to those stressors, and telomere length in immune cells.

With 2 months of daily data on child-reported parent–child conflict (described above) we could compute an individual's average parent–child conflict exposure over a 2-month period. Additionally, we had measures of child-reported parent–child warmth (e.g., "My mom/dad and I got along well today"), marital conflict (e.g., "My Mom and Dad argued today"), and marital affection ("My Mom and Dad kissed or hugged today"). Thus, we could assess exposure to conflict and warmth in the family environment. With daily reports of negative and positive mood (example items are: sad, on edge; relaxed, happy, respectively), we computed associations between exposures (conflict, warmth) and mood for each child across 2 months by generating empirical Bayes' estimates in multilevel modeling (Cohen, Doyle, & Skoner, 1999; Mohr et al., 2013). These "reactivity scores," represented conceptually on the left side of Fig. 8.3 reflected the association between an exposure measure (e.g., parent–child warmth) and mood (positive mood). We then tested two different models of how family environments might impact telomere length, where the dependent variable of interest was children's immune cell telomere length at the end of the study: an "exposure" model that used average levels of parent–child and marital conflict and warmth as predictors, and a "reactivity" model that used reactivity scores as predictors. A conceptual description of the analytic approach is shown at the right portion of Fig. 8.3, and the primary finding is shown in bold. Specifically, children who tended to report greater negative affect on days that they also reported greater marital conflict showed lower immune cell telomere length, even after controlling for average levels of conflict and warmth. Our findings are consistent with models of biological embedding of childhood adversity (Miller, Chen, & Parker, 2011), as well as models linking family environments to emotional reactivity and health (Repetti et al., 2011; Troxel & Matthews, 2004), and were made possible by intensive repeated measures over multiple days.

In this "first derivative" application, the inference is that intensive repeated measures provide a metric of a child's potential to respond to marital conflict with negative mood. However, our daily diary approach places some key boundary conditions on that metric. A stronger association between marital conflict and negative mood in some children compared to others may also indicate that some children are more likely to recall marital conflict when they are in a negative mood (mood-congruent recall), or that certain children that report more daily negative affect may promote interparental conflict (Kihlstrom, Eich, Sandbrand, & Tobias, 2000; Schermerhorn, Chow, & Cummings, 2010). Disentangling "reactivity" from mood-congruent recall or stress generation requires frequent sampling used in ecological momentary assessment approaches and is a key direction for future work.

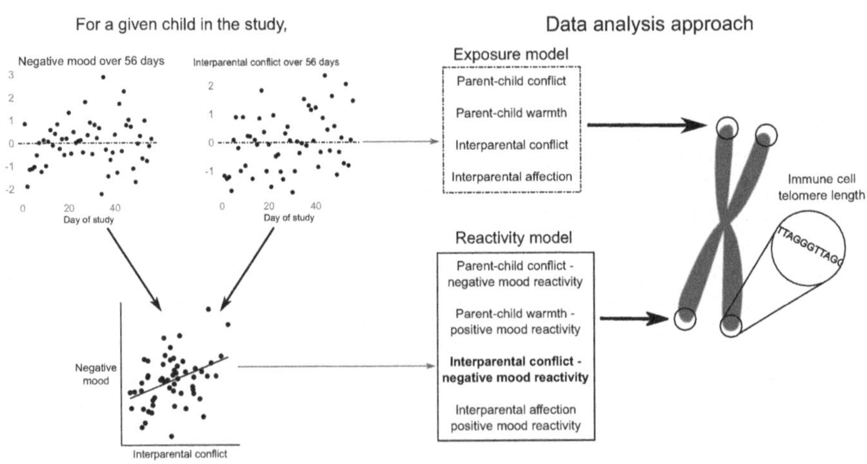

Fig. 8.3 Conceptual depiction of reactivity scores (left), and data analyses linking daily conflict/ warmth in the family environment to immune cell telomere length

8.2.2 Using Genomic Approaches to Conceptualize the Potential to Respond to Infectious Threats

Thus far, "first derivative" has been represented by within-person changes in a variable over time, or within-person changes in one variable (mood) as a function of within-person changes in another psychological variable (conflict and warmth). Both approaches were made possible through intensive repeated measures over time, which could be extended to allostatic biological processes, such as cardiovascular, neuroendocrine, or immune function. However, intensive repeated measures of biological processes can be burdensome, highly invasive, and intrusive. Thus, biobehavioral researchers have been exploring "snapshot" measures that can provide more than just a snapshot—that is, single-occasion measures that may provide a window into first derivatives of biological functioning. Importantly, while those snapshot measures can provide inferences about how biological systems normally function, they are not used to infer anything about psychological states or stress exposures. One area of significant interest in biobehavioral research, with applications across a number of psychological phenomena and health problems that includes assessing "potential" to respond, is the body's rapid immune response to infection and injury: inflammation (Kiecolt-Glaser, McGuire, Robles, & Glaser, 2002).

The immune system's primary job is to recognize threats to the organism like viruses and bacteria and respond to those threats by eliminating them (for accessible reviews, see Repetti et al., 2011; Robles, Glaser, & Kiecolt-Glaser, 2005). The initial immune response to threat, whether that be bacteria invading through a cut, or viruses infecting the cells that line one's nasal cavity, involves a rapid response from immune cells which produce chemical messengers that can disrupt the ability of viruses and bacteria to function, recruit additional help by increasing blood flow to the affected site and attracting other immune cells, and activate other immune cells to respond. Immune cells also "eat" and break down foreign particles when possible. Taken together, inflammation is the rapid immune response to infection and injury, and has taken on significant prominence in biobehavioral research because inflammation: (1) plays a key role in the pathophysiology of chronic conditions considered major public health threats including cardiovascular disease and Alzheimer's disease; (2) is a key player in ubiquitous health conditions like upper respiratory infections; and importantly, (3) is influenced by and influences social and emotional functioning (Kiecolt-Glaser et al., 2002; Robles et al., 2005).

Multiple cells drive the inflammatory response, and for simplicity I focus on a particular immune cell—the macrophage—which is also called a monocyte when it circulates in blood (Owen, Punt, & Stranford, 2013). Macrophages/monocytes inhabit most tissues in the body, and are important sentinels in tissues that interface with the outside environment, like the skin, lungs, and gut (Geissmann et al., 2010). Within a single macrophage (shown in Fig. 8.4), the inflammatory response is initiated when the macrophage detects a threat through specially designed "detectors" known as toll-like receptors. When the detector is activated, such as through binding

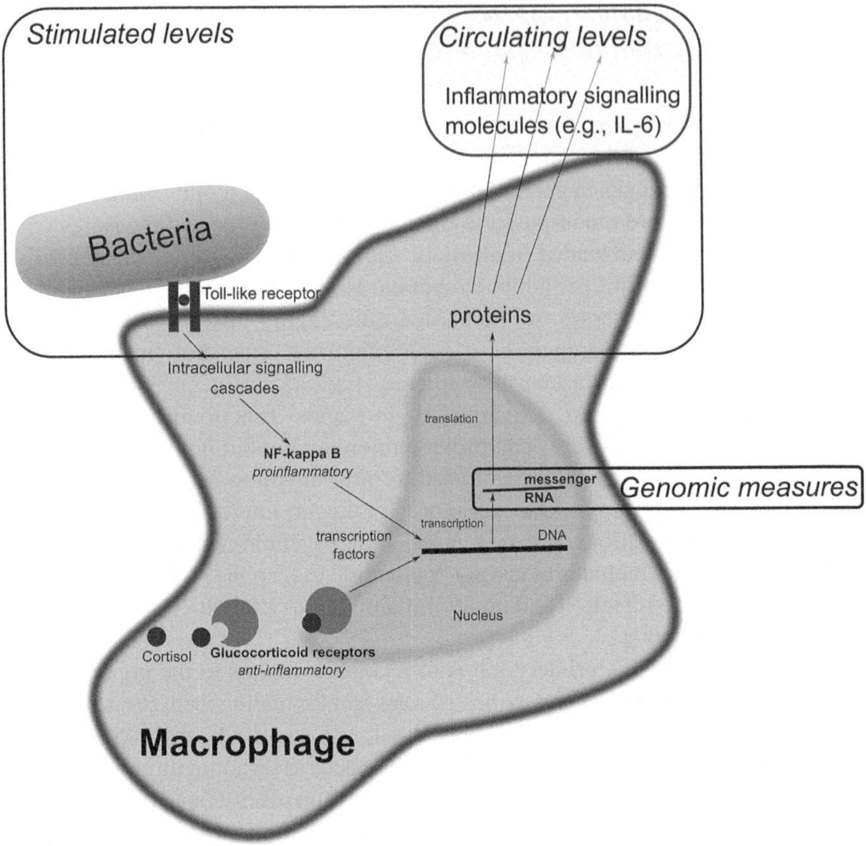

Fig. 8.4 Diagram of the inflammatory response at the level of a single macrophage, with measures of inflammation shown in the rounded rectangles

to a bacteria, this sets off a cascade of signals within the macrophage that ultimately lead to the activation of nuclear factor kappa B (NF-κB), which is a "transcription factor" molecule that migrates into the nucleus of the macrophage (Cole, Yan, Galic, Arevalo, & Zack, 2005). Transcription factors are generally responsible for activating specific genes within a cell, leading to the transcription of those genes into messenger RNA (mRNA), and the eventual translation of that mRNA into protein. In the context of inflammation, NF-κB migrates to the cell nucleus, leading to transcription of genes that code the chemical messengers that are involved in the inflammatory response. Thus, conceptually speaking indicators of greater NF-κB activation also indicate that the inflammatory response is either turned on or has greater potential to be turned on. Figure 8.4 also indicates that other intracellular processes that are involved in turning off inflammation and highlights the glucocorticoid receptor. When cortisol binds to the glucocorticoid receptor, the complex travels to the nucleus and inhibits the transcription of inflammation-related genes. In sum, NF-κB is widely viewed as a key *pro*-inflammatory transcription factor, and the glucocorticoid receptor is viewed as a key *anti*-inflammatory transcription factor.

Figure 8.4 also describes the multiple methods (described in *italics*) that exist for measuring the inflammatory response. The primary methods are measuring circulating levels of inflammatory biomarkers from blood; or removing immune cells from blood, stimulating those cells with molecules that initiate an inflammatory response (i.e., lipopolysaccharide, which is the main component of the cell wall of certain types of bacteria), and measuring inflammatory biomarkers produced inside immune cells or secreted outside the cell (Vedhara & Wang, 2005). Each measure has strengths and limitations, and the goal here is to focus on the degree to which such measures can be used as measures of potential to respond to infectious threats. Conceptually, measuring potential to respond to threats requires knowing measuring "the threat" (exposure) and the response to the threat. Circulating measures of inflammatory biomarkers provide a window into responses, but not exposures. Stimulating immune cells involves deliberately exposing cells to a threat and measuring the response, making stimulated measures the most ideal. However, stimulated inflammatory responses pose logistical challenges that are particularly problematic to family and developmental researchers. Namely, blood must be transported immediately to the laboratory for processing (isolating cells) and stimulation, and immunology laboratories often operate according to normal business hours (i.e., 8 am to 5 pm on weekdays). Thus, drawing blood from children and families during times that are convenient and minimally intrusive, such as evenings and weekends, may not be feasible for an immunology laboratory. Thus, the most ideal method for assessing potential to respond may not be logistically possible in family research.

Genomic approaches to studying the inflammatory response, with a focus on the transcription factor control pathways described above, may provide a feasible but somewhat imperfect window into first derivative approaches to the inflammatory response. Such methods involve determining gene expression through sequencing mRNA in immune cells and making inferences about what genes are being expressed, the function of those genes, and potential themes inherent in the patterns of gene expression (Cole, 2010, 2014). Transcription factors are one possible theme; researchers can ask whether genes regulated by NF-κB or GR appear to be differentially active in people with differing levels of exposure to a psychosocial factor of interest. Notably, exposure to stressful events that including caregiving for brain cancer patients (Miller et al., 2014), chronic interpersonal stress (Miller, Rohleder, & Cole, 2009), and exposure to the combination of low SES and low levels of maternal warmth in childhood (Chen, Miller, Kobor, & Cole, 2011) are all related to greater expression of pro-inflammatory genes regulated by NF-κB and lower expression of anti-inflammatory genes regulated by GR.

We sought to extend prior work on social adversity and inflammation-related gene expression to conflict and warmth in the family environment, and importantly, examine patterns in children and their parents (Robles et al., 2018). In addition, to take advantage of the multi-method (interview, questionnaire, and daily diary) and multi-reporter (parents and children) approach to assessing the family environment, we combined measures of family conflict across methods and reporters (see Robles et al., 2018 for more details). Similar to the telomere work described above, whole blood was obtained from parents and children who elected to provide samples. Following RNA extraction from immune cells, we used gene microarray technology to quantify expression of over 30,000 genes in immune cells.

For parents and children separately, we compared patterns of gene expression between participants in high vs. low conflict families, which yielded lists of several hundred differentially (over- and under-) expressed genes. The gene lists were analyzed by a bioinformatics tool that allowed for inferring whether genes regulated by the transcription factors NF-κB and GR were relatively over- or under-expressed in high conflict/low warmth families (Cole et al., 2005). For both children and parents, living in a high conflict family was associated with greater expression of genes regulated by NF-κB, consistent with the pro-inflammatory phenotype observed in prior work. Parents, but not children, in high conflict families also showed lower expression of genes regulated by GR, consistent with the idea that chronic stress may lead to immune cells becoming insensitive to the effects of cortisol. Interestingly, for children, greater family conflict was related to more upper respiratory infection symptoms, both on days when children were not verifiably "sick" with the cold or flu, and on days when children had verifiable illness. The latter provides an example of a potential clinical consequence of a pro-inflammatory phenotype. In sum, our gene expression data provide a potential "first derivative" window into how the immune system might respond to threats as a function of the family environment. Both parents and children in higher conflict family environments may have more amplified inflammatory responses to threats that activate the immune system, and there may be clinical consequences as well, such as more severe upper respiratory infection symptoms.

8.3 Implications

8.3.1 Implications for Practice and Policy

Our work highlights the importance of including intensive repeated measures to monitor mechanisms of change (e.g., preventing increases in conflict over time, reducing negative mood reactivity to conflict). For instance, repeated assessments of family functioning over time can provide a window into the speed of progress in family-based treatments. Moreover, repeated assessments of family functioning and mood may provide insight into the degree to which family interventions can "loosen" the ties between stressors at home and mood. For instance, a plausible treatment target in family therapy may be reducing the covariation between interparental conflict and children's mood, so that interparental conflict becomes less distressing over time and children understand that disagreements between spouses/partners are normative (assuming a healthy level of conflict exists in the interparental relationship). Our work also provides insight into biomarkers that may be responsive to interventions (and downstream health outcomes plausibly linked to those downstream mediators), such as bedtime cortisol; such biomarkers may be useful secondary outcomes for use in efficacy and effectiveness trials. However, the value of collecting biomarkers for the purpose of monitoring children and families during interventions in everyday clinical practice has not been demonstrated; this remains a key issue for future effectiveness down the road.

Research on intensive repeated measures and genomic markers of risk, such as pro-inflammatory gene expression, is still in very early phases. Thus, translating research from the initial studies described in this chapter may be a bit premature. That said, work on biobehavioral research on families and resilience more generally suggests several implications for policy and program evaluation. Programs and policies that are specifically designed to intervene at the level of family, including financial or instrumental assistance, or increasing access to family-based interventions for families at risk, should consider including measures of the quality of the family environment as primary outcomes, and health outcomes as secondary outcomes. In addition, recent efforts to include assessments of the social environment, including experiencing recent stressors, and degree of social integration into electronic health records may be extended to assessments of conflict and warmth in the family environment. Finally, given the implications of chronic inflammation for current and long-term health, systemic levels of circulating inflammatory biomarkers or perhaps even "first derivative" measures of inflammatory response potential may be considered as exploratory outcomes in family-based interventions to reduce risk and increase resilience.

8.3.2 Implications for Understanding Family Resilience

This chapter described several examples of how understanding exposures using intensive repeated measures provides insight into the biobehavioral mechanisms that may be sensitive to the family environment, including HPA axis regulation, immune cell aging, and inflammation, and that have biologically plausible health implications can be conceptualized based on how intensive repeated measures change over time, such as increases in conflict over several weeks to months, or increases in support and involvement, respectively. Perhaps more intriguing is using relationships between frequently sampled measures, such as greater or lower emotional reactivity to daily interparental conflict, to conceptualize risk or resilience. On the one hand, conceptualizations of risk/resilience that focus on individual differences in capacity to respond in better or worse ways to adversity may be interested in using the covariation between two measures as ways to identify individuals who are "at risk" (e.g., high, positive within-person correlation between conflict and negative mood) or "resilient" (e.g., high, positive within-person correlation between family support and positive mood). On the other hand, prevention and intervention research that focuses on reducing risk and increasing resilience may examine covariation between two measures as ways to evaluate treatment mechanisms or efficacy. For instance, if family therapy can reduce the within-person correlation between interparental conflict and children's negative mood from pre- to post-treatment, this could be a mechanism of treatment effects or even an indicator of treatment outcomes.

On the biological side, incorporating minimally invasive and logistically feasible measures that indicate how a person may respond to physical threats like infection or other immune-stimulating substances like environmental pollutants, with sensitive measures of stress exposure in the family environment, are a key future direction for research on family risk and resilience. Individuals who have known exposures to physical threats, like high frequency of infections or living in regions with high pollution exposure, may be key populations to explore the deleterious effects of stressful family environments. In addition, individuals who have high pro-inflammatory phenotype potential may be a key subgroup for whom family-based prevention and intervention research is indicated.

8.4 Conclusions

I conclude this chapter by emphasizing the need for replication of the effects described in this chapter, particularly in samples with large sample sizes with longitudinal follow-up. At the same time, the research described herein provides "proof-of-concept" for the value of incorporating intensive sampling of the naturalistic family environment in future biobehavioral research. In addition, the work described in this chapter complements other theory and research that emphasizes the key role of inflammation and the regulation of inflammation in linking risk and resilience in families to current and future physical health (Kiecolt-Glaser et al., 2002; Miller, Chen, & Cole, 2009; Repetti et al., 2011). Family therapists and researchers recognized long ago that families are dynamic entities; research methodologies that capture the dynamic ebb and flow within families over time, as well as the internal dynamics of how the family environment regulates immunity, will be key tools in understanding family risk and resilience in the decades to come.

Questions for Thought and Discussion

1. What are some of the potential challenges to using biomarkers in our study of stress and health? How do we mitigate those challenges and collect high-quality biological and physiological data?
2. What insights does the HPA axis give us into the physiological and emotional well-being of individuals? What might it tell us about an individual's surroundings, relationships, or other life circumstances?
3. The immune system is another critical biological system. What is the relationship between stress and immune system function? What are some of the consequences to the immune system from stressful life events?

4. What is inflammation? What is its contribution to physical health and emotional functioning?
5. What are the potential health risks, both physical and emotional, associated with long-term exposure to a high conflict/low warmth family environment? How might family-level relational interventions benefit the physical health of family members?

Glossary

Allostatic Processes Biological changes designed to help organisms adapt to changes in the environment, including changes in the cardiovascular, neuroendocrine, and immune systems.

Biological Mediators Biological systems and processes that can explain links between psychosocial factors and health.

Cortisol A glucocorticoid hormone produced in the adrenal cortex, in response to signals from the brain as part of the hypothalamic-pituitary-adrenal axis; frequently measured in naturalistic settings in saliva; plays a critical role in regulating metabolism and immune function.

Genomics Studying biological processes using genetic material, including messenger ribonucleic acid (mRNA), and the patterns of gene expression from that material.

Hypothalamic-Pituitary-Adrenal (HPA) Axis A major neuroendocrine system that plays a key role in allostatic processes.

Immune System Responsible for recognizing and responding to threats inside the organism; composed of numerous cells, tissues, and organs, as well as signaling molecules.

Inflammation The body's first line of immune defense against infection and injury; also described as innate immunity.

Intensive Repeated Measures Psychosocial assessments that are administered with a high degree of frequency over long periods of time.

Macrophage/Monocyte Key cell involved in innate immunity that produces inflammatory responses.

Nuclear Factor Kappa B A transcription factor that regulates the activation of genes within immune cells that promote inflammation.

Telomere Nucleotide structures at the end of chromosomes that protect genetic material from being damaged during the process of normal cell division; shorten with each cell division.

Transcription The process by which genetic code in deoxyribonucleic acid (DNA) is read and coded into messenger RNA; the first part of the central dogma of molecular biology.

Translation The process by which mRNA is read and coded into amino acids, which are then assembled into proteins; the second part of the central dogma of molecular biology.

References

Biomarker Definitions Working Group. (2001). Biomarkers and surrogate endpoints: Preferred definitions and conceptual framework. *Clinical Pharmacology and Therapeutics, 69*, 89–95. https://doi.org/10.1067/mcp.2001.113989

Blackburn, E. H. (2000). Telomere states and cell fates. *Nature, 408*(6808), 53–56. https://doi.org/10.1038/35040500

Cacioppo, J. T., & Tassinary, L. G. (1990). Inferring psychological significance from physiological signals. *American Psychologist, 45*, 16–28. https://doi.org/10.1037/0003-066x.45.1.16

Campisi, J., & di Fagagna, F. D. A. (2007). Cellular senescence: When bad things happen to good cells. *Nature Reviews Molecular Cell Biology, 8*, 729–740. https://doi.org/10.1038/nrm2233

Charles, S. T., Piazza, J. R., Mogle, J., Sliwinski, M. J., & Almeida, D. M. (2013). The wear and tear of daily stressors on mental health. *Psychological Science, 24*, 733–741. https://doi.org/10.1177/0956797612462222

Chen, E., Miller, G. E., Kobor, M. S., & Cole, S. W. (2011). Maternal warmth buffers the effects of low early-life socioeconomic status on pro-inflammatory signaling in adulthood. *Molecular Psychiatry, 16*, 729–737. https://doi.org/10.1038/mp.2010.53

Cohen, S., Doyle, W. J., & Skoner, D. P. (1999). Psychological stress, cytokine production, and severity of upper respiratory illness. *Psychosomatic Medicine, 61*, 175–180.

Cole, S. W. (2010). Elevating the perspective on human stress genomics. *Psychoneuroendocrinology, 35*, 955–962. https://doi.org/10.1016/j.psyneuen.2010.06.008

Cole, S. W. (2014). Human Social Genomics. *PLoS Genet, 10*, e1004601. https://doi.org/10.1371/journal.pgen.1004601

Cole, S. W., Yan, W., Galic, Z., Arevalo, J., & Zack, J. A. (2005). Expression-based monitoring of transcription factor activity: The TELiS database. *Bioinformatics, 21*, 803–810. https://doi.org/10.1093/bioinformatics/bti038

Davies, P. T., & Cummings, E. M. (1994). Marital conflict and child adjustment: An emotional security hypothesis. *Psychological Bulletin, 116*, 387–411. https://doi.org/10.1037/0033-2909.116.3.387

Davies, P. T., & Martin, M. J. (2013). The reformulation of emotional security theory: The role of children's social defense in developmental psychopathology. *Development and Psychopathology, 25*, 1435–1454. https://doi.org/10.1017/s0954579413000709

Drury, S. S., Mabile, E., Brett, Z. H., Esteves, K., Jones, E., Shirtcliff, E. A., & Theall, K. P. (2014). The association of telomere length with family violence and disruption. *Pediatrics, 134*, E128–E137. https://doi.org/10.1542/peds.2013-3415

Geissmann, F., Manz, M. G., Jung, S., Sieweke, M. H., Merad, M., & Ley, K. (2010). Development of monocytes, macrophages, and dendritic cells. *Science, 327*(5966), 656–661. https://doi.org/10.1126/science.1178331

Harkness, K. L., & Monroe, S. M. (2016). The assessment and measurement of adult life stress: Basic premises, operational principles, and design requirements. *Journal of Abnormal Psychology, 125*, 727–745. https://doi.org/10.1037/abn0000178

Kiecolt-Glaser, J. K., McGuire, L., Robles, T. F., & Glaser, R. (2002). Emotions, morbidity, and mortality: New perspectives from psychoneuroimmunology. *Annual Review of Psychology, 53*, 83–107. https://doi.org/10.1146/annurev.psych.53.100901.135217

Kihlstrom, J. F., Eich, E., Sandbrand, D., & Tobias, B. A. (2000). *Emotion and memory: Implications for self-report*. Mahwah, NJ: Erlbaum.

Kuhlman, K. R., Repetti, R. L., Reynolds, B. M., & Robles, T. F. (2016). Change in parent-child conflict and the HPA-axis: Where should we be looking and for how long? *Psychoneuroendocrinology, 68*, 74–81. https://doi.org/10.1016/j.psyneuen.2016.02.029

Lehman, B. J., & Repetti, R. L. (2007). Bad days don't end when the school bell rings: The lingering effects of negative school events on children's mood, self-esteem, and perceptions of parent-child interaction. *Social Development, 16*, 596–618. https://doi.org/10.1111/j.1467-9507.2007.00398.x

Lippold, M. A., McHale, S. M., Davis, K. D., Almeida, D. M., & King, R. B. (2016). Experiences with parents and youth physical health symptoms and cortisol: A daily diary investigation. *Journal of Research on Adolescence, 26*, 226–240. https://doi.org/10.1111/jora.12186

Miller, G. E., & Chen, E. (2010). Harsh family climate in early life presages the emergence of a proinflammatory phenotype in adolescence. *Psychological Science, 21*, 848–856. https://doi.org/10.1177/0956797610370161

Miller, G. E., Chen, E., & Cole, S. W. (2009). Health psychology: Developing biologically plausible models linking the social world and physical health. *Annual Review of Psychology, 60*, 501–524. https://doi.org/10.1146/annurev.psych.60.110707.163551

Miller, G. E., Chen, E., & Parker, K. J. (2011). Psychological stress in childhood and susceptibility to the chronic diseases of aging: Moving toward a model of behavioral and biological mechanisms. *Psychological Bulletin, 137*, 959–997. https://doi.org/10.1037/a0024768

Miller, G. E., Murphy, M. L. M., Cashman, R., Ma, R., Ma, J., Arevalo, J. M. G., … Cole, S. W. (2014). Greater inflammatory activity and blunted glucocorticoid signaling in monocytes of chronically stressed caregivers. *Brain Behavior and Immunity, 41*, 191–199. https://doi.org/10.1016/j.bbi.2014.05.016

Miller, G. E., Rohleder, N., & Cole, S. W. (2009). Chronic interpersonal stress predicts activation of pro- and anti-inflammatory signaling pathways 6 months later. *Psychosomatic Medicine, 71*, 57–62. https://doi.org/10.1097/PSY.0b013e318190d7de

Mohr, C. D., Brannan, D., Wendt, S., Jacobs, L., Wright, R., & Wang, M. (2013). Daily mood-drinking slopes as predictors: A new take on drinking motives and related outcomes. *Psychology of Addictive Behaviors, 27*, 944–955. https://doi.org/10.1037/a0032633

Mukherjee, S. (2015). *The gene: An intimate history*. New York, NY: Simon & Schuster.

Owen, J. A., Punt, J., & Stranford, S. (2013). *Kuby immunology*. New York, NY: Freeman.

Puterman, E., & Epel, E. (2012). An intricate dance: Life experience, multisystem resiliency, and rate of telomere decline throughout the lifespan. *Social and Personality Psychology Compass, 6*, 807–825. https://doi.org/10.1111/j.1751-9004.2012.00465.x

Repetti, R. L. (1996). The effects of perceived daily social and academic failure experiences on school-age children's subsequent interactions with parents. *Child Development, 67*, 1467–1482. https://doi.org/10.1111/j.1467-8624.1996.tb01808.x

Repetti, R. L., Reynolds, B. M., & Sears, M. S. (2015). Families under the microscope: Repeated sampling of perceptions, experiences, biology, and behavior. *Journal of Marriage and Family, 77*, 126–146. https://doi.org/10.1111/jomf.12143

Repetti, R. L., Robles, T. F., & Reynolds, B. (2011). Allostatic processes in the family. *Development and Psychopathology, 23*, 921–938. https://doi.org/10.1017/S095457941100040X

Reynolds, B. M., Robles, T. F., & Repetti, R. L. (2016). Measurement reactivity and fatigue effects in daily diary research with families. *Developmental Psychology, 52*, 442–456. https://doi.org/10.1037/dev0000081

Robles, T. F., & Carroll, J. E. (2011). Restorative processes and health. *Social and Personality Psychology Compass, 5*, 518–537. https://doi.org/10.1111/j.1751-9004.2011.00368.x

Robles, T. F., Carroll, J. E., Bai, S., Reynolds, B. M., Esquivel, S., & Repetti, R. L. (2016). Emotions and family interactions in childhood: Associations with leukocyte telomere length. *Psychoneuroendocrinology, 63*, 343–350. https://doi.org/10.1016/j.psyneuen.2015.10.018

Robles, T. F., Glaser, R., & Kiecolt-Glaser, J. K. (2005). Out of balance: A new look at chronic stress, depression, and immunity. *Current Directions in Psychological Science, 14*, 111–115. https://doi.org/10.1111/j.0963-7214.2005.00345.x

Robles, T. F., Repetti, R. L., Reynolds, B. M., Chung, P. J., Arevalo, J. M., & Cole, S. W. (2018). Family environments and leukocyte transcriptome indicators of a proinflammatory phenotype in children and parents. *Development and Psychopathology, 30*, 235–253. https://doi.org/10.1017/S0954579417000591

Robles, T. F., Reynolds, B. M., Repetti, R. L., & Chung, P. J. (2013). Using daily diaries to study family settings, emotions, and health in everyday life. *Journal of Social and Personal Relationships, 30*, 179–188. https://doi.org/10.1177/0265407512457102

Schermerhorn, A. C., Chow, S. M., & Cummings, E. M. (2010). Developmental family processes and interparental conflict: Patterns of micro level influences. *Developmental Psychology, 46*, 869–885. https://doi.org/10.1037/a0019662

Shalev, I. (2012). Early life stress and telomere length: Investigating the connection and possible mechanisms. *Bioessays, 34*, 943–952. https://doi.org/10.1002/bies.201200084

Shalev, I., Moffitt, T. E., Sugden, K., Williams, B., Houts, R. M., Danese, A., … Caspi, A. (2013). Exposure to violence during childhood is associated with telomere erosion from 5 to 10 years of age: A longitudinal study. *Molecular Psychiatry, 18*, 576–581. https://doi.org/10.1038/mp.2012.32

Slatcher, R. B., & Robles, T. F. (2012). Preschoolers' everyday conflict at home and diurnal cortisol patterns. *Health Psychology, 31*, 834–838. https://doi.org/10.1037/a0026774

Slopen, N., McLaughlin, K. A., & Shonkoff, J. P. (2014). Interventions to improve cortisol regulation in children: A systematic review. *Pediatrics, 133*, 312–326. https://doi.org/10.1542/peds.2013-1632

Troxel, W. M., & Matthews, K. A. (2004). What are the costs of marital conflict and dissolution to children's physical health? *Clinical Child and Family Psychology Review, 7*, 29–57. https://doi.org/10.1023/B:CCFP.0000020191.73542.b0

Ulrich-Lai, Y. M., & Herman, J. P. (2009). Neural regulation of endocrine and autonomic stress responses. *Nature Reviews Neuroscience, 10*, 397–409. https://doi.org/10.1038/nrn2647

Vasan, R. S. (2006). Biomarkers of cardiovascular disease. *Molecular Basis and Practical Considerations, 113*, 2335–2362. https://doi.org/10.1161/circulationaha.104.482570

Vedhara, K. V., & Wang, E. C. Y. (2005). Assessment of the immune system in human psychoneuroimmunology. In K. V. Vedhara & M. R. Irwin (Eds.), *Human psychoneuroimmunology* (pp. 53–80). London, UK: Oxford University Press. https://doi.org/10.1093/med:psych/9780198568841.003.0003

Index

A. W. Harrist, B. C. Gardner (eds.), *Biobehavioral Markers in Risk and Resilience Research*, Emerging Issues in Family and Individual Resilience,
https://doi.org/10.1007/978-3-030-05952-1

The manufacturer's authorised representative in the EU is Springer Nature Customer Service Centre GmbH, Europaplatz 3, 69115 Heidelberg, Germany. If you have any concerns regarding our products, please contact ProductSafety@springernature.com

Printed and bound by CPI Group (UK) Ltd, Croydon, CR0 4YY
22/09/2026
02221061-0019